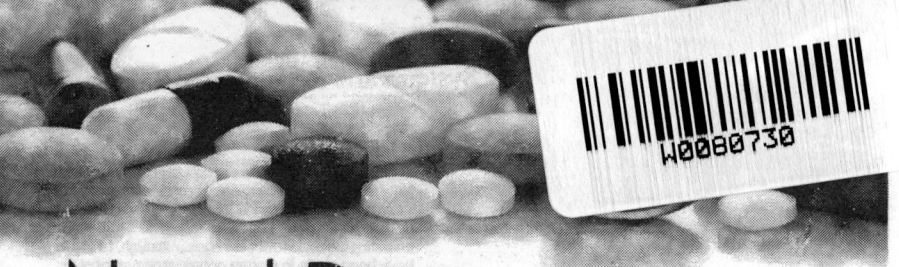

Novel Drug Delivery Systems and Regulatory Affairs

Basavaraj K Nanjwade M Pharm PhD

Professor
Department of Pharmaceutics
KLE University's College of Pharmacy
Belgaum
Karnataka, India

V Sai Kishore M Pharm PhD

Associate Professor
Department of Pharmaceutics
Bapatla College of Pharmacy
Bapatla
Andhra Pradesh, India

Sachin A Thakare M Pharm PGDMM

Department of Pharmaceutics
KLE University's College of Pharmacy
Belgaum
Karnataka, India

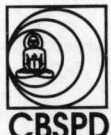

CBSPD

CBS Publishers & Distributors Pvt Ltd

New Delhi • Bengaluru • Chennai • Kochi • Kolkata • Lucknow• Mumbai
Hyderabad • Jharkhand • Nagpur • Patna • Pune • Uttarakhand

Novel Drug Delivery
Systems and
Regulatory Affairs

ISBN: 978-93-88527-45-3

CBS Reprint: 2019, 2024
First Edition: 2011

Published by Satish Kumar Jain and Produced by Varun Jain for

CBS Publishers & Distributors Pvt Ltd
4819/XI Prahlad Street, 24 Ansari Road, Daryaganj, New Delhi 110 002, India.   4819/XI Prahlad Street, 24 Ansari Road, Daryaganj, New Delhi 110 002, India.
Ph: 23289259, 23266861   Website: www.cbspd.com
                                            e-mail: delhi@cbspd.com
Corporate Office: 204 FIE, Industrial Area, Patparganj, Delhi 110 092
Ph: 011-4934 4934   Fax: 011-4934 4935   e-mail: publishing@cbspd.com;
                                            publicity@cbspd.com

Branches

- **Bengaluru:** Seema House 2975, 17th Cross, K.R. Road, Banasankari 2nd Stage, Bengaluru 560 070, Karnataka
  Ph: +91-80-26771678/79   Fax: +91-80-26771680   e-mail: bangalore@cbspd.com
- **Chennai:** 7, Subbaraya Street, Shenoy Nagar, Chennai 600 030, Tamil Nadu, India
  Ph: +91-44-26680620/26681266   Fax: +91-44-42032115   e-mail: chennai@cbspd.com
- **Kochi:** 42/1325, 1326, Power House Road, Opp KSEB, Power House, Ernakulam 682 018, Kochi, Kerala, India
  Ph: +91-484-4059061-65, 67   Fax: +91-484-4059065   e-mail: kochi@cbspd.com
- **Kolkata:** 147, Hind Ceramics Compound, 1st Floor, Nilgunj Road, Belghoria, Kolkata-700056, West Bengal, India
  Ph: +033-25633055, 033-25633056   e-mail: kolkata@cbspd.com
- **Lucknow:** Basement, Khushnuma Complex, 7 Meerabai Marg (Behind Jawahar Bhawan), Lucknow-226001, UP, India
  Ph: +91-522-4000032   e-mail: tiwari.lucknow@cbspd.com
- **Mumbai:** PWD Shed, Gala no 25/26, Ramchandra Bhatt Marg, Next to JJ Hospital Gate no. 2, Opp. Union Bank of India Noorbaug, Mumbai-400009, Maharashtra, India
  Ph: 022-66661880/89   e-mail: mumbai@cbspd.com

Representatives

• **Hyderabad**	0-9885175004	• **Jharkhand**	0-9811541605	• **Nagpur**	0-8692091830
• **Patna**	0-9334159340	• **Pune**	0-9664372571	• **Uttarakhand**	0-9716462459

Printed at Glorious Printers, Delhi, India

Preface

In recent year the pharmaceutical technology has undergone a many changes with the development of New techniques of method of preparation and testing pharmaceutical and changes in regulatory affairs, with these development pharmaceutical education has also seen many changes.

The purpose of this text book is to introduce pharmacy students to the basic systems of pharmaceutical principles and technologies applied in preparation of various Novel drug delivery systems and introduction to the regulatory agencies and Current Good Manufacturing Practices (cGMP).

With the changing trends in pharmaceutical education at higher levels the Pharmacy Council of India (PCI) according to ER.1991 has revised the course contents for Degree pharmacy students to bring their knowledge up-to-date.

There are many textbook available on the subject, but the material in most of them is presented in a diffused form or in highly specialized and discernible to those in the pharmacy field. The major objective of writing this book is to present the information in a simple language style and lucid has been kept to help the student to grasp the subject and understand easily. The subject matter is covered in accordance with the prescribed syllabus for this course. The diagram are neatly drawn, adequately labelled and given wherever they are needed. The revision question has been given at the end of textbook to enable the student the confident about the subject.

The book has 8 Units and the greater emphasis is on Advances in Novel Drug Delivery and Regulatory affairs. Thus an attempt has been made to provide most consolidate and up-to-date information on different topics which is a time consuming.

It is hoped that this book will also well received both by the teachers and students. Any suggestion and comments for further improvement of the book from teacher and students are most welcome and will be deeply appreciated and thankfully acknowledged.

The authors express their sincere thanks and appreciation to Prof. Dr. F. V. Manvi Principal and Prof. Ashok D. Taranalli Vice Principal, KLE University College of Pharmacy, Belgaum. Also to Prof. Dr. Chandrakant K. Kokate Vice-Chancellor and Prof. Dr. P. F. Kotur Registrar, KLE University, Belgaum, Karnataka, India for rendering useful suggestions and inputs, apart from being intensely persuasive to complete the project.

We are grateful to Mr. Gowrishetty Madhusudhan IKON BOOKS publication who has taken keen interest and spared no pains for the fine getup of book.

Authors

Table of Contents

Chapter 4 Targeted Drug Delivery Systems

Chapter 5 Narcotic Drugs and Psychotropic Substances Act 1985 and A.P.N.D.P.S Rules1986

Chapter 6 Quality Assurance

Chapter 7 Good manufacturing practices

Chapter 8 Introduction to Validation

Chapter 1

ORAL CONTROLLED DRUG DELIVERY SYSTEM

1.1 INTRODUCTION

The development of controlled-release formulations continues to be a big success for the pharmaceutical industry. The success of any technology relies on the ease of its manufacturing process and its reproducibility of desirable biopharmaceutical properties. The optimal design of controlled release systems (CRDs) necessitaties a thorough understanding of pharmacodynamic and pharmacokinectics of drugs. The primary objective of controlled drug deliveryis to ensure safety and improve the efficacy of drug as well as patients compliance through better control of plasma drug level and less frequent dosing.

"An ideal controlled drug delivery system is the one which delivers the drug at a predetermined rate, locally or systemically, for a specified period of time" The basic objective of controlled drug delivery system is to optimize the pharmacokinectics, biopharmaceutics and pharmacodynamic properties of drug in such a way that its utility is maximized through reduction in side effect and cure or control of condition in the shortest possible time by using smallest quantity of drug administered by most suitable route.

Controlled release technology is evolved with matrix technology several articles in the 1950s and 1960s reported simple matrix tablets or monolithic granules. In 1952 Smith Kline & French introduced the spansule a time release formulation that launched a wide spread search for the other application in the design of dosage forms.

1.2 ORAL CONTROLLED DRUG DELIVERY SYSTEM

Oral routes has been the commonly adopted, the most popular and has received more attention in the pharmaceutical field because of convenience of ease of administration, more flexibility in the designing of dosage forms than the drug delivery design for other routes, ease of production and low cost of such a system. The oral drug delivery depends on various factors such as type of delivery system, the disease being treated, the patient, the length of the therapy and properties of the drug. The controlled release system for the oral use are mostly solids and based on dissolution, diffusion or a combination of both mechanisms in the control of release rate of drug. The physico-chemical properties include solubility crystal nature, partition coffecient, intrinsic dissolution etc dosage form characteristic are controlled and optimized with respect to physicochemical properties of drug and relevant GI environment factors. The other to be considered are diseased state, the patient compliance and duration of therapy. The goal of targeted oral drug delivery system is to achieve better therapeutic success compared to conventional dosage form of same drug. This could be achieved by improving the pharmacokinectics profile, patient convenience and compliance in therapy.

ADVATAGES OF ORAL CONTROLLED RELEASE DRUG DELIVERY

➢ Improved patient compliance: improved patient compliance is due to, reduced frequency of administration.

➢ Reduced side effects: reduced side effects is due to, low dose.

➢ Less fluctuating plasma drug level: less fluctuating plasms drug level is maintained with controlled drug delivery systems, because the drug is slowly released from the dosage form continuously and maintains the constant blood level, where as in case of immediate release dosage form, the plasma level was raised immediately, once the Cmax is reached it will fall down, if we take the dose again the concentration will be raised up, it is fluctuating, whereas in case of controlled drug delivery system, constant plasma level is maintained.

➢ Better stability of drug.

1.3 CLASSIFICATION OF ORAL CONTROLLED RELEASE DRUG DELIVERY SYSTEM

On the basis of mechanism of drug release the oral system are classified as follows:-

> Dissolution controlled release.

> Diffusion controlled release.

> Ion exchange resins.

> pH Independent systems.

> Osmotically controlled release.

> Altered density formulation/ Buoyant systems.

A) DISSOLUTION CONTROLLED RELEASE

These system are easiest to design. The drug with slow dissolution rate is inherently sustained for e.g griseofulvin, digoxin and salycilamide such drugs act as natural prolonged release products others such as aluminium aspirin, ferrous sulfate, and benzphetamine paomate, produce slow dissolving form when it comes in contact with GI fluids. And drugs having high aqueous solubility and dissolution rate e.g pentoxifylline. Steriod have been reported to undergo transformation into less soluble polymorphs during dissolution in absorption pool.

The basic principle of dissolution control is as follows: If the dissolution process is diffusion layer controlled where the rate of diffusion from the solid surface through a unstirred liquid film to the bulk solution is rate limiting the flux is 'J' is given by

$J = -D(dc/dx)$

Where,

D = diffusion cofficient.

Dc/dx = concentration gradeint between the solid surface and bulk of solution.

In terms of flow rate of material (dm/dt) through unit area (A), the flux can be given as

$$J = (1/A) \, dm/dt$$

For the system with linear concentration gradient and thickness of the diffusion layer 'h'

$$dc/dx = (Cb - Cs)$$

Where Cs represents the concentration at the solid surface and Cb is the bulk solution concentration. A combined equation for rate of material is given as

$$dm/dt = - (DA/h) \, (Cb - Cs) = kA \, (Cs - Cb)$$

Where, k is intrinsic dissolution rate constant.

The above equation predicts constants dissolution rate if the surface area, diffusion coefficient, diffusion layer thickness, and concentration difference are kept constant. However, as dissolution proceeds, all of the parameters, the surface area especially, may change.

Dissolution controlled release products are divided in two clases:

1) Encapsulation dissolution control.

2) Matrix dissolution control.

1) Encapsulation/ Coating dissolution controlled system (Reservoir Devices)

Encapsulation involves coating of individual particles, or granules of drug with the slowly dissolving material. The particles obtain after coating can be compressed directly into tablets as in spacetabs or placed in capsules as in the spansule products. The drug release is controlled by dissolution rate of polymeric coat. As the time required for dissolution of coat is a function of its thickness and the aqueous solubility of the polymer one can obtain the coated particles of varying thickness in the range of 1- 200 micron. By using one of several microencapsulation techniques the drug particles are coated or encapsulated with slowly dissolving materials like cellulose, PEGs, polymethacrylates, waxes etc.

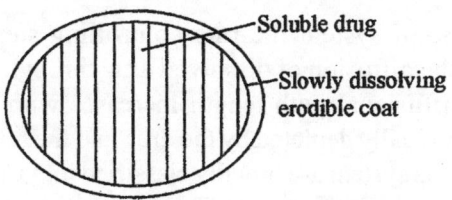

Fig.1: Encapsulation/ Coating dissolution controlled system
(Reservoir Devices)

2) Matrix (or Monolith)/ Embedded dissolution controlled system.

Since the drug is homogeneously dispersed throughout a rate controlling medium matrix system are also called monoliths. The waxes used for such system are beeswax, carnauba wax, hydrogenated castor oil etc. These waxes control the drug dissolution by controlling the rate of dissolution fluid penetration into the matrix by altering the porosity of tablet, decreasing its wettability or by itself dissolved at a slower rate. The dispersion of drug wax is prepared by dispersing the drug in the molten wax followed by congealing and granulating the same. The process, compression parameters and size of particles formed determine the release rate from this system. The drug release is often first order from such matrices.

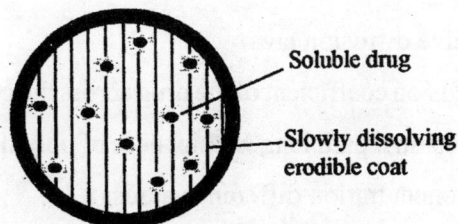

Fig.2: Matrix (or Monolith)/ Embedded dissolution
controlled system.

A) DIFFUSION CONTROLLED RELEASE SYSTEM

In these type of system the rate controlling step is not the dissolution rate but the diffusion of dissolved drug through a polymeric barrier. Since the diffusional path length increases with time as the insoluble matrix is gradually depleted by the drug and the release of drug is never zero order. This system are broadly classified into two categories reservoir system and monolithic system. The mechanism of both system is quiet different.

B) RESERVOIR DEVICES (OR LAMINATED MATRIX DEVICES)

These system are hollow in which core of drug is surrounded in water insoluble polymer membrane. Coating or microencapsulation technique are used to apply polymer. The permeability of membrane depend on the thickness of the coat/concentration of coating solution and on the nature of polymer HPC, ethylcellulose, and polyvinyl acetate are the commonly used polymer in such devices. The mechanism of drug release across the membrane involves partitioning into the membrane with subsequent release into the surrounding fluid by diffusion. The rate of drug release from the reservoir system can be explained by Ficks Law of diffusion.

$$dm/dt = DSK(\ddot{A}C)/l$$

Where,

S = is the active diffusion area.

D = is the diffusion coefficient of the drug across the coating membrane.

l = is the diffusional path length (thickness of polymer coat)

$\ddot{A}$C = is the concentration difference across l.

K = is the partition coefficient of the drug between polymer and the external medium.

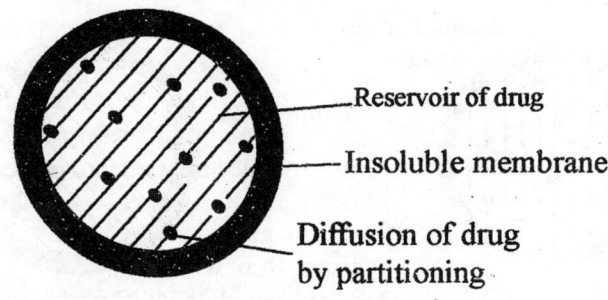

Reservoir of drug

Insoluble membrane

Diffusion of drug
by partitioning

Fig.3: Reservoir Devices (or Laminated matrix devices)

C) MATRIX DIFFUSION CONTROLLED SYSTEM

In these system the drug is dispersed in insoluble matrix of rigid non swellable hydrophobic materials or swellable hydrophillic substances. Insoluble plastics such as PVC and fatty materials like stearic acid, beeswax etc are the material used for rigid matrix. The drug is generally kneaded within the solution of plastic material such as PVC in an organic solvent and granulated. The wax drug matrix is prepared by dispersing the drug in molten fat followed by congealing. The release of highly water soluble drug can be sustained by using swellable matrix systems. Hydrophillic gums and may be of natural origin (guar, gum, tragacanth), semisynthetic (HPMC, CMC, Xanthan gum) or synthetic (polyacrylamides) are the material generally used for such matrices. In the solvent such as alcohol the gum and drug are granulated together and compressed into tablet. The mechanism of drug release from these system involve initial dehydration of hydrogel which involves absorption of water and desorption of drug via swelling controlled diffusion mechanism. As the gum swells and the drug diffuses out of it, the swollen mass devoid of drug appear transparent or glass like and therefore the system is sometimes called as glassy hydrogel.

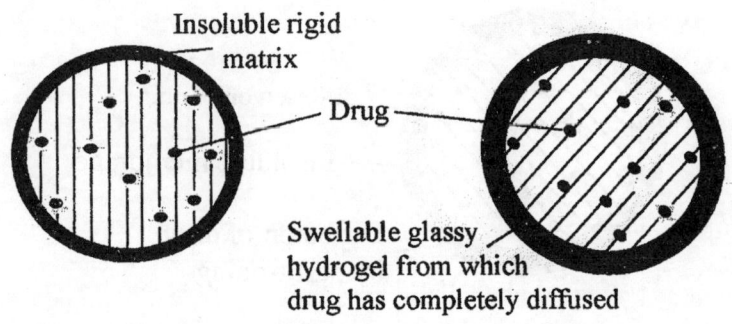

Insoluble rigid matrix

Drug

Swellable glassy hydrogel from which drug has completely diffused

Fig.4: MATRIX DIFFUSION CONTROLLED SYSTEM

1.4 ION EXCHANGE RESIN

Ion exchange resin(IER) have received considerable attention from pharmaceutical scientists because of their versatile properties as drug delivery vehicles. Over the last few years research has revealed that IER are equally suitable for drug delivery technologies, including controlled release, transdermal, nasal, topical and taste masking. Dose dumping is the major drawback of sustained release of extended release or extended release, resulting in increased risk of toxicity. Because of their better drug-retaining properties and prevention of dose dumping the use of IER has occupied an important place in the development of controlled- or sustained-release systems. Synthetic ion exchange resins have been used in pharmacy and medicine for taste masking or controlled release of drug. Drug resin complexation converts drug to amorphous form leading to improved drug dissolution. Several studies have reported the use of IER for drug delivery at the desired site of action. Sulfonated and carboxylic resins with a polystyrene backbone are most widely used in clinical medicine.

Ion exchange resins are cross-linked, water insoluble, polymer-carrying, ionizable functional groups. Drugs can be loaded onto the resins by an exchanging reaction, and hence, a drug-resin complex (drug resinate) is formed. The drug is released from the resinates by exchanging with ions in the gastrointestinal fluid, followed by drug diffusion. Being high molecular weight water insoluble polymers, the resins are not absorbed by the body and are therefore inert. It is an attractive method for sustained release drug delivery systems. Drug release characteristics depend upon the ionic environment of the resin containing drug. Therefore, it is less susceptible to environment conditions such as enzyme content and pH at the absorption site. This approach requires the presence of ions in solution, and therefore it would not be applicable to the skin, or other areas with limiting quantities of eluting ions. This approach requires the presence of ions in solution, and therefore it would not be applicable to the skin, or other areas with limiting quantities of eluting ions.

MECHANISM AND PRINCIPLE

Resins are water-insoluble materials containing anionic or cationic groups in repeating units on the resin chain. Anion-exchange resin involve basic functional groups (usually a polyamine) capable of removing anions from acidic solutions. An Anion Exchange Resin generally has quaternary ammonium groups and polyalkylamine functional groups as an integral part of the resin and an equivalent amount of anionic drug molecules. Cation-exchange resins contain acidic functional groups.

A Cation Exchange Resin generally has Sulphonic and Carboxylic functional groups as an integral part of the resin and an equivalent amount of cationic drug molecules. Although their exact composition may vary, they usually contain polystyrene polymer with either sulfonic, carboxylic or phenolic groups.

Cation exchange resin

$$H^+ + Resin - SO_3 \cdot Drug^+ \rightleftharpoons Resin - SO_3 \cdot H^+ + Drug^+$$

Anion exchange resin

$$Cl^- + Resin - N(CH_3)_3^+ Drug^- \rightleftharpoons Resin - N(CH_3)_3^+ Cl^- + Drug^-$$

$Resin - SO_3 \cdot H^+$ represents cation exchange resin & $Resin - N(CH_3)_3^+$ represents anion exchange. $Drug^+$ is basic drug and $Drug^-$ is acidic drug. Ion exchange resonates when administered resides two hours in the stomach in contact with acidic fluid pH 1.2 and then move to the intestine where they remain in contact for more than 6 hours with a alkaline fluid.

Types of Drug Resin Interactions

Electrostatic interaction

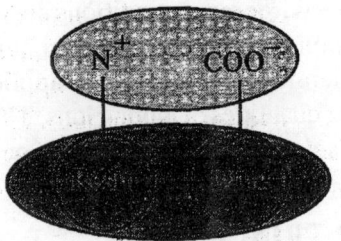

Hydrophobic interaction

Fig.5: Electrostatic and hydrophobic interaction seen in drug resin complex

Types of Ion Exchange Resins

There are two major classes of ion exchange polymers cation-exchanger, whose functional groups can undergo reaction with cations of a surrounding solution and anion exchangers whose functional groups can undergo reaction with the anions of surrounding solution.

Resin type	Chemical constitution	Structure
Strongly acidic cation exchanger	Sulphonic acid group attached to a styrene and divinylbenzene copolymer	$R - SO_3 \cdot H^+$
Weakly acidic cation exchanger	Carboxylic acid group attached to an acrylic and divinylbenzene copolymer	$R - COO \cdot Na^+$
Strongly basic anion exchanger	Quaternary ammonium group attached to a styrene and divinylbenzene copolymer	$R -N (CH_3)_3{}^+ Cl^-$
Weakly basic anion exchanger	Polyalkylamine group attached to a styrene and divinylbenzene copolymer	$R -NH (R)_2{}^+ Cl^-$

Drugs Suitable for Resinate Preparation

1. Drugs should have acidic and basic groups in their chemical structure.

2. Biological half life should be between 2-6 hrs, drugs with $t_{1/2}$ < 1 hr or > 8 hrs are difficult to formulate.

3. The drug is to be absorbed from all regions of GI tract.

4. Drugs should be stable sufficiently in the gastric juice.

ADVANTAGES OF RESIN

1. Resins being polyelectrolytes have extensive binding sites leading to very high drug loading ability.

2. They are chemically inert and free from local and systemic side effects.

3. Because of ion exchange ability, they have been used in taste masking, modified release and therapeutic applications.

4. All conventional solid, semisolid and liquid dosage forms can be prepared by using resins.

5. They have been used in selective separation/recovery of pharmaceuticals from mixtures.

6. Being stable to all sterilization means, can be formulated in to all sterile dosage forms.

Ion Activated Drug delivery system.

An ionic or charged drug can be delivered by ion-activated drug delivery system. It is prepared by first complexing an ionic drug with an ion exchange resin containing a suitable counter ion. (cationic drug with $SO3^-$, anionic drug with $N(CH3)3^+$).

The granules of drug resin complex was first treated with an impregnating agent, PEG-4000, to reduce the rate of swelling in an aqueous environment and then coated by air suspension coating, with a water insoluble polymer such as ethyl cellulose. This membrane serve as a rate controlling barrier to modulate the in flux of ion as well as the release of drug from the system. In electrolyte medium, such as gastric fluid, ions diffuse in to system, react with drug-resin complex and trigger the release of ionic drug. This system is exemplified by the development of pennkinetic, which permits the formulation of liquids suspension dosage form with sustain release drug properties for oral administration. Since GI fluid regularly maintains a constant level of ions, theoretically the delivery of drug from this ion activated oral drug delivery system can be maintain at the relatively constant rate.

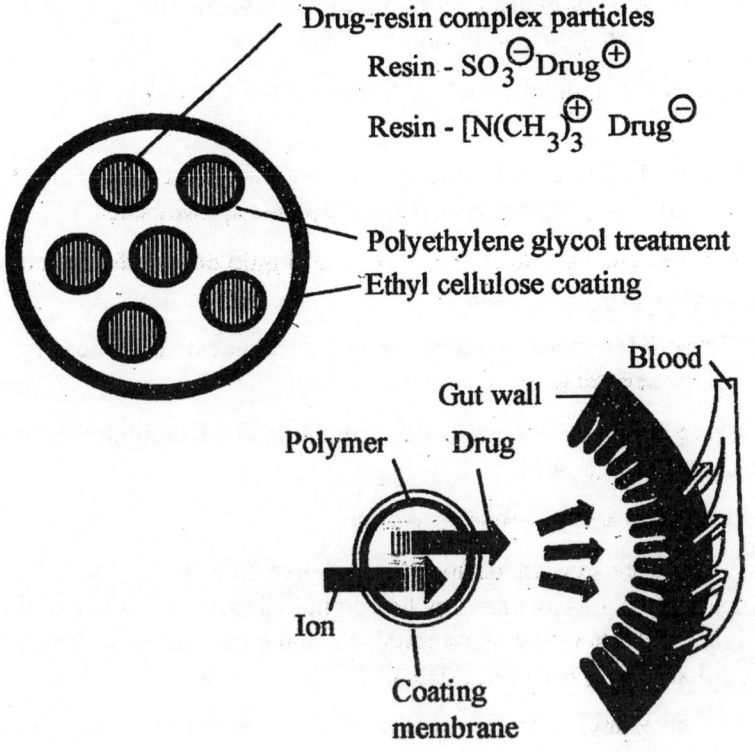

Fig.6: Ion Activated Drug delivery system.

1.5 OSMOTIC CONTROLLED DRUG DELIVERY SYSTEM

A number of design options are available to control or modulate the drug release from a dosage form. Majority of per oral dosage form fall in the category of matrix, reservoir or osmotic system. In matrix system, the drug is embedded in polymer matrix and the release takes place by partitioning of drug into the polymer matrix and the release medium. In contrast, reservoir systems have a drug core surrounded\coated by the rate controlling membrane. However factor like pH, presence of food and other physiological factor may affect drug release from conventional controlled release systems. Osmotic systems utilize the principle of osmotic pressure for the delivery of drugs. Drug release from these systems is independent of pH and other physiological parameter to a large extent and it is possible to modulate the release characteristic by optimizing the properties of drug and system. The oral osmotic pumps have certainly came a long way and the available products on this technology and number of patent granted in the last few years makes it presence felt in the market. They are also known as gastro intestinal therapeutic system. Alza corporation of the USA was first to develop an oral osmotic pump and today also they are the leaders in this field with a technology named OROS (Osmotic drug delivery).

Osmosis

Osmosis refers to the process of movement of solvent molecules from lower concentration to higher concentration across a semi permeable membrane. Osmosis is the phenomenon that makes controlled drug delivery a reality. Osmotic pressure created due to imbitions of fluid from external environment into the dosage form regulates the delivery of drug from osmotic device. Rate of drug delivery from osmotic pump is directly proportional to the osmotic pressure developed due to imbitions of fluids by osmogen. Osmotic pressure is a colligative property of a solution in which the magnitude of osmotic pressure of the solution is independent on the number of discrete entities of solute present in the solution. Hence the release rate of drugs from osmotic dispensing devices is dependent on the solubility and molecular weight and activity coefficient of the solute (osmogent).

Osmotic pressure is used as driving force for these systems to release the drug in controlled manner. Osmotic drug delivery technique is the most interesting and widely acceptable among all other technologies used for the same.

Principle

In osmotic drug delivery system osmotic pressure is the driving force that generates constant drug release. In this system the drug reservoir can be solution or a solid formulation and is placed within the semi permeable housing with controlled water permeability. The drug is activated to release in solution form at a constant rate through a special delivery orifice.

For the drug delivery system containing solution formulation the intrinsic rate of release Q/t is given by,

$$Q/t = P_w A_m / h_m \ (\eth_s - \eth_e)$$

If the drug delivery system is solid so the intrinsic rate of drug release Q/t is given by:

$$Q/t = P_w A_m / h_m \ (\eth_s - \eth_e) \ S_d$$

Where, Pw = water permeability.

Am = effective surface area.

hm = thickness of the semipermiable housing.

(+"s- +"e) = deferential osmotic pressure b/w drug delivery system and external environment.

Sd = aqueous solubility of the drug contained in solid formulation.

Release of drug is activated by osmotic pressure and controlled at a rate deyermined by water permeability, effective surface area of semi permeable housing and osmotic pressure gradient.

Eg: Acutrim, an oral rate controlled drug delivery system is solid tablet of water soluble and osmotically active phenylpropanolamine (PPA) Hcl enclosed wthin a semipermeable membrane made from cellulose triacetate. Semi permeable layer is further coated with PPA for immediate release. In GIT, GI fluids will dissolve immediately releasable layer, which provides initial dose and its water components then penetrates through the semipermeable at the rate determined by $P_w A_m / h_m$ dissolve the controlled release dose of PPA under osmotic pressure differential created $(\delta_s - \delta_e)$, the PPA solution is delivered at a controlled rate through an orifice predrilled by laser beam. It is designed to provide a controlled delivery of PPA for duration of 16hr for appetite suppression in weight control program.

Basic Component Of Osmotic Pumps

1. Drug.

2. Osmotic agent.

3. Semi permeable membrane.

1.DRUG

Drug with short biological half-life {2-6hr}

· Highly potent drug

· Required for prolonged treatment

e.g. nifedipine, glipizide, virapamil.

2. OSMOTIC AGENT

Osmogents used for fabrication of osmotic dispensing device are inorganic or organic in nature a water soluble drug by it self can serve the purpose of an osmogent.

Inorganic water-soluble osmogents:

Magnesium sulphate.

Sodium chloride.

Sodium sulphate.

Potassium chloride.

Sodium bicarbonate.

Organic polymer osmogents:

    Sodium carboxymethyl cellulose.

    Hydroxypropylmethyl cellulose.

    Hydroxyethylmethylcellulose.

    Methylcellulose.

    Polyethylene oxide.

    Polyvinyl pyrollidine.

List of some osmotic agents with their osmotic pressure

Compound	Osmotic pressure(atm)
Sodium chloride	356
Fructose	355
Potassium chloride	245
Sucrose	150
Dextrose	82
Mannitol	3

3. SEMI PERMEABLE MEMBRANE

    The semi permeable membrane should be a stable both to the outer inner environment of the device. The membrane must be sufficiently rigid so as to retain its dimensional integrity during the operational lifetime of the device. The membrane should also be relatively impermeable to the contents of dispenser so that osmogent is not lost by diffusion across the membrane finally, the membrane must be biocompatible

Ideal Property of Semi Permeable Membrane

    The Semi Permeable Membrane must meet some performance criteria

1. The material must posses sufficient wet strength (-10^5) and wet modulus so as to retain its dimensional integrity during the operational lifetime of the device.

2. The membrane exhibit sufficient water permeability so as to retain water flux rate in the desired range. The water vapor transmission rates can be used to estimate water flux rates

3. The reflection coefficient and leakiness of the osmotic agent should approach the limiting value of unity. Unfortunately, polymer membranes that are more permeable to water are also, in general more permeable to the osmotic agent.

4. The membrane should also be biocompatible.

A) Oral osmotic pumps

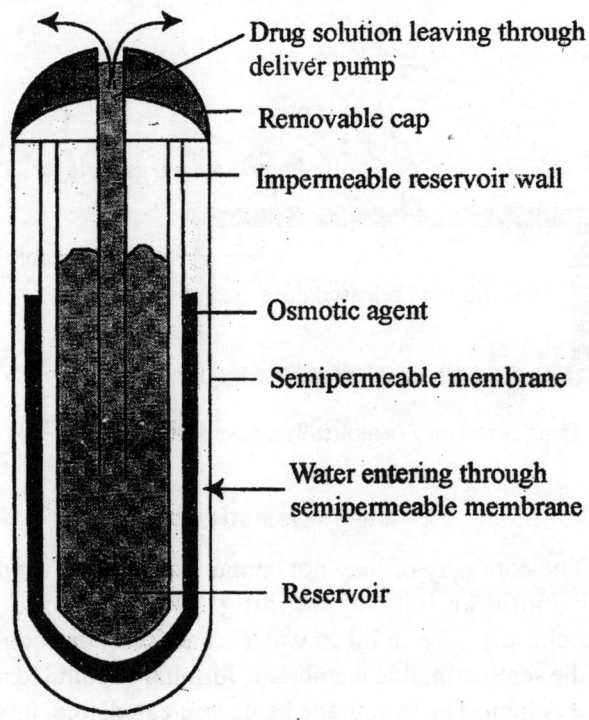

Fig.7: Oral osmotic pumps

There are two types of pumps:

1) Single chamber osmotic pump.

   a) Elementary osmotic pump

2) Multi chamber osmotic pump.

   a) Push pull osmotic pump.

   b) Osmotic pump with non expanding second chamber.

3) Elementary osmotic pump.

It is simplest possible form of osmotic pump as it does not require special equipment and technology. It can be mass –produced economically using ordinary tabletting and coating machine and a facility to drill an orifice.

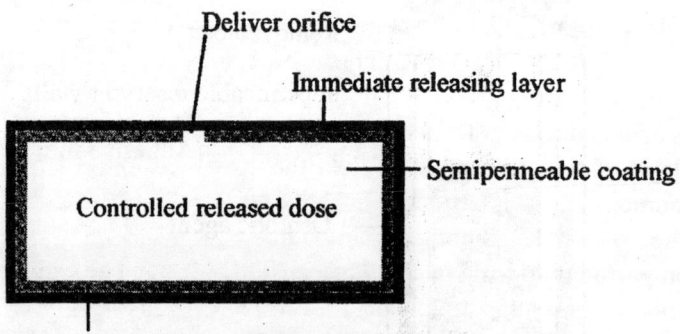

Fig.8: Osmotic pump

The core may or may not contain an osmotic agent depending on the osmotic activity of the drug. When exposed to aqueous environment, the core imbibes water osmotically at a controlled rate through the semipermiable membrane, forming a saturated drug solution inside the system. The membrane being non-extensible, internal volume of the pump remains constant. The system delivers, via the orifice, in any time interval, a volume of saturated solution of drug equal to volume of water uptake. This process is continues at a constant rate until all solid drug inside the tablet has been dissolved and only a solution filled shell remains. The residual dissolved drug continues to be delivered, but at a declining rate, until the osmotic pressure inside and outside the pump is equal. These system are suitable or delivery of drugs having moderate water solubility.

B) Push pull osmotic pump.

Push pull osmotic pump is a modified Elementary osmotic pump. (EOP). through, which it is possible to deliver both poorly water-soluble and highly water soluble drugs at a constant rate. This system resembles a standard bilayer coated tablet. One layer (depict as the upper layer) contains drug in a formulation of polymeric, osmotic agent and other tablet excipients. This polymeric osmotic agent has the ability to form a suspension of drug in situ. When this tablet later imbibes water, the other layer contains osmotic and colouring agents, polymer and tablet excipients. These layer are formed and bonded together by tablet compression to form a single bilayer core. The tablet core is then coated with semipermeable membrane. After the coating has been applied, a small hole is drilled through the membrane by a laser or mechanical drill on the drug layer side of the tablet. When the system is placed in aqueous environment water is attracted into the tablet by an osmotic agent in both the layers. The osmotic attraction in the drug layer pulls water into the compartment to form in situ a suspension of drug. The osmotic agent in the non-drug layer simultaneously attract water into that compartment, causing it to expand volumetrically and the expansion of non drug layer pushes the drug suspension out of the delivery orifice.

C) Osmotic pump with non expanding second chamber.

The second category of multi-chamber devices comprises system containing a non-expanding second chamber. This group can be divided into two sub groups, depending on the function of second chamber. In one category of these devices, the second chamber is used to dilute the drug solution leaving the devices. This is useful because in some cases if the drug leaves the oral osmotic devices a saturated solution, irritation of GI tract is a risk.

Example:- the problem that lead to withdrawal of osmosin, the device consist of a normal drug containing porous tablet from which drug is released as a saturated solution. However before the drug can escape from the device it must pass through a second chamber. Water is also drawn osmotically into this chamber either because of osmotic pressure of drug solution or because the second chamber contain, water soluble diluents such as NaCl. This type of devices consist of two rigid chamber, the first chamber contains a biologically inert osmotic agent, such as sugar or a simple salt like sodium chloride, the second chamber contains the drug. In use water is drawn into both the chamber through the surrounding semi permeable membrane. The solution of osmotic agent formed in the first chamber then passes through the connecting hole to the drug chamber where it mixes with the drug solution before exiting through the micro porous membrane that form a part of wall surrounding the chamber. The device could be used to deliver relatively insoluble drugs.

D) Osmotic Brusting Osmotic Pump

This system is similar to an Elementary osmotic pump(EOP) expect delivery orifice is absent and size may be smaller. When it is placed in an aqueous environment, water is imbibed and hydraulic pressure is built up inside until the wall rupture and the content are released to the environment. Varying the thickness as well as the area the semipermeable membrane can control release of drug. This system is useful to provide pulsated release.

Advantage

Osmotic drug delivery system for oral and parenteral use offer distinct and practical advantage over other means of delivery. The following advantages contributed to the popularity of osmotic drug delivery system.

1. They typically give a zero order release profile after an initial lag.

2. Deliveries may be delayed or pulsed if desired.

3. Drug release is independent of gastric pH and hydrodynamic condition.

4. They are well characterized and understood.

5. The release mechanisms are not dependent on drug.

6. A high degree of in-vitro and in vivo correlation

7. The rationale for this approach is that the presence of water in g.i.t. is relatively constant, at least in terms of the amount required for activation and controlling osmotically base technologies.

Disadvantage

1 Costly.

2. If the coating process is not well controlled there is a risk of film defects, which results in dose dumping.

3. Size hole is critical.

Marketed Products

Product Name	Active	Design	Dose
Acutrim	Phenylpropanolamine	Elementary pump	75 mg
Alpress LP	Prazosin	Push -Pull	2.5 - 5 mg
Cardura XL	Doxazosin	Push -Pull	4, 8 mg
Covera HS	Verapamil	Push -Pull with time delay	180, 240 mg
Ditropan XL	Oxybutinin chloride	Push -Pull	5, 10 mg
Dynacirc CR	Isradipine	Push -Pull	5, 10 mg
Efidac 24	Pseudoephiderine	Elementary Pump	60 mg IR, 180 mg CR
Efidac 24	Chlorpheniramine meleate	Elementary Pump	4 mg IR, 12 mg CR
Glucotrol XL	Glipizide	Push - Pull	5, 10 mg

1.6 ALTERED DENSITY (Floating systems or Hydrodynamically controlled systems)

Floating systems or Hydrodynamically controlled systems are low-density systems that have sufficient buoyancy to float over the gastric contents and remain buoyant in the stomach without affecting the gastric emptying rate for a prolonged period of time. While the system is floating on the gastric contents, the drug is released slowly at the desired rate from the system. After release of drug, the residual system is emptied from the stomach. This results in an increased GRT and a better control of the fluctuations in plasma drug concentration. However, besides a minimal gastric content needed to allow the proper achievement of the buoyancy retention principle, a minimal level offloating force (F) is also required to keep the dosage form reliably buoyant on the surface of the meal.Many buoyant systems have been developed based on granules, powders, capsules, tablets, laminated films and hollow microspheres. These considerations have led to the development of oral floating dosage forms possessing gastric retention capabilities. Thus when a drug possesses a narrow 'absorption window' design of sustained release preparation require both prolongation of gastrointestinal transit time of dosage forms and controlled drug release.

Basic Gastrointestinal Tract Physiology

Anatomically the stomach is divided into 3 regions: fundus, body, and antrum (pylorus). The proximal part made of fundus and body acts as a reservoir for undigested material, whereas the antrum is the main site for mixing motions and act as a pump for gastric emptying by propelling actions. Gastric emptying occurs during fasting as well as fed states. The pattern of motility is however distinct in the 2 states. During the fasting state an interdigestive series of electrical events take place, which cycle both through stomach and intestine every 2 to 3 hours.14 This is called the interdigestive myloelectric cycle or migrating myloelectric cycle (MMC), which is further divided into following 4 phases as described

1. Phase I (basal phase) lasts from 40 to 60 minutes with rare contractions.

2. Phase II (preburst phase) lasts for 40 to 60 minutes with intermittent action potential and contractions. As the phase progresses the intensity and frequency also increases gradually.

3. Phase III (burst phase) lasts for 4 to 6 minutes. It includes intense and regular contractions for short period. It is due to this wave that all the

undigested material is swept out of the stomach down to the small intestine. It is also known as the housekeeper wave.

4. Phase IV lasts for 0 to 5 minutes and occurs between phases III and I of 2 consecutive cycles.

After the ingestion of a mixed meal, the pattern of contractions changes from fasted to that of fed state. This is also known as digestive motility pattern and comprises continuous contractions as in phase II of fasted state. These contractions result in reducing the size of food particles (to less than 1 mm), which are propelled toward the pylorus in a suspension form. During the fed state onset of MMC is delayed resulting in slowdown of gastric emptying rate. Scintigraphic studies determining gastric emptying rates revealed that orally administered controlled release dosage forms are subjected to basically 2 complications, that of short gastric residence time and unpredictable gastric emptying rate.

1.7 SELECTION OF DRUG CANDIDATE

> Drug which are predominantly absorbed from the upper part of GIT.
> Drug that are acting locally in stomach.
> Drugs those are poorly soluble at alkaline pH.
> Drugs that degrade in the colon.

Eg: Cholrpheniramine maleate, Theophylline, Furosemide,

Ciprofloxacin, Captopril, Acetylsalicylic acid, Nimodipine,

Amoxycillin trihydrate, Verapamil HCI, Isosorbide di nitrate, Sotalol, Isosorbide mononitrate, Aceraminophen, Ampicillin, Cinnarazine, Dilitiazem, Florourracil,

Piretanide, Prednisolone.

Major requirement for Floating drug delivery system

> It must form a cohesive gel barrier.
> Specific gravity lower than gastric content(1.004 – 1.010g/cc)
> Release content slowly to serve as reservoir.

20 – 75% w/w of one or more gel forming hydrocolloid are incorporated in to the formulation and then compressing these granules into a table t(or encapsulating into capsules)

Eg : Hydroxyethyl cellulose.

    Hydroxypropyl cellulose

    Hydroxypropyl methyl cellulose.

    Sodium carboxy methyl cellulose.

Types of Floating drug delivery system.

1. Effervescent system.

2. Non-effervescent system.

Effervescent system

    Floatability can be achieved by generation of gas bubbles. CO_2 can be generated in situ by incorporation of carbonates or bicarbonates, which react with acid either the natural gastric acid or co-formulated as citric or tartaric acid.

    These floating drug delivery system employes matrices from swelling polymers like methocel or chitosan and effervescent components such as sodium bicarbonate and tartaric or citric acid or matrices having a chambers of liquid components that gasify at body temperature. The matrices are prepared in such manner that when they come in contact with stomach fluid, carbon di oxide is generated and retained entrapped in hydrocolloid gel. This leads to an upward flow of dosage form and maintains its floating condition.

    A single layered tablet can be prepared by initially mixing the carbon dioxide generating the components in tablet matrix. A bilayered tablet may be compressed in which the gas liberating component is present in hydrocolloid layer and the drug is compressed in other layer for sustained release.

Non Effervescent system

    Non-effervescent floating dosage forms use a gel forming or swellable cellulose type of hydrocolloids, polysaccharides, and matrix-forming polymers like polycarbonate, polyacrylate, polymethacrylate, and polystyrene. The formulation method includes a simple approach of thoroughly mixing the drug and the gel-forming hydrocolloid. After oral administration this dosage form swells in contact with gastric fluids and attains a bulk density of G<1. The air entrapped within the swollen matrix imparts buoyancy to the dosage form. The so formed swollen gel-like structure acts as a reservoir and allows sustained release of drug through the gelatinous mass.

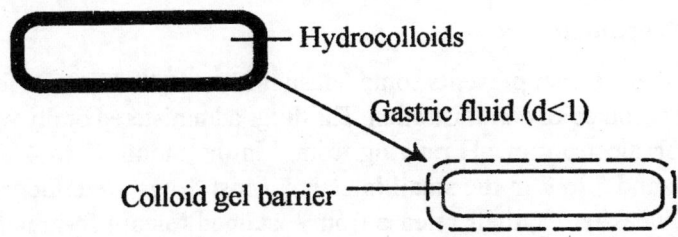

Hydrocolloids

Gastric fluid (d<1)

Colloid gel barrier

Fig.9: Mechanism of Non Effervescent system

ADVANTAGES:

1. Improved Drug absorption, because of increase GRT and more time spent by the dosage form at its absorption site.

2. Controlled delivery of drugs

3. Delivery of the drug for local action in stomach

4. Minimizing the mucosal irritation due to the drugs, by drug releasing slowly at controlled rate.

5. Treatment of Gastrointestinal disorders such as gastro-esophageal reflux

6. Simple and conventional equipments required for manufacture

7. Ease of administration and better patient compliance,

8. Site specific drug delivery

DISADVANTAGES

1. Floating system is not feasible for those drugs that have solubility or stability problem in G.I. tract.

2. These systems require a high level of fluid in the stomach for drug delivery to float and work efficiently coat, water.

3. The drugs that are significantly absorbed through out gastrointestinal tract, which undergo significant first pass metabolism, are only desirable candidate.

pH Independent

The GI tract presents some unusual features that are not found in the other routes of administration. The drugs administered orally would encounter spectrum of pH ranging from 7 in the mouth, 1 to 4 in the stomach, and 5 to 7 in the small intestine. Most drugs are either weak acids or weak bases, their release from sustained release formulations is pH dependent.

Eg: papaverine hydrochloride was release in the gastric region than in the intestine because of its higher solubility in the upper part of the GI tract.

Buffers can be added to the formulation the maintain a constant pH thereby rendering the pH independent drug release. Salts of amino acids, citric acids, phthalic acid, phosphoric acid or tartaric acid are commonly used because of their physiological accecpectibility. The rate of availability of propoxyphene from a buffered controlled release formulation showered significantly increased reproducibility. The granules are design for oral controlled release of basic or acidic drug at a rate i.e independent of pH in the GI tract. They are prepared by mixing a basic or acidic drug with one or more buffering agents, granulating with appropriate pharmaceutical excipients, and finally, coating with a gastrointestinal fluid permeable film-forming polymer. When the GI fluid permeates through the membrane, the buffering agents adjust the fluid inside to a suitable constant pH, thereby rendering a constant rate of drug release.

REVIEW QUESTIONS

ESSAY QUESTIONS

1. How does Controlled Drug Delivery system differs from conventional and sustained release systems and Write Advantages and Disadvantages of controlled release preparations?

2. What factors should be considered in the design of a Controlled Drug Delivery system and What criteria are necessary for selection and exclusion of drug as a candidate for Controlled Drug Delivery system?

3. List the physicochemical and biological properties of drug and state pharmacokinetic and pharmacodynamic parameters are important in the design of controlled release formulations?

4. Explain the concepts /approaches for osmotic based systems?

5. Enumerate the properties of pH independent systems and What are various ways by which controlled drug release through altered density systems can be obtained?

6. What criteria should be followed in polymer selection for Controlled Drug Delivery and write classification and the applications of polymers?

7. What are objectives of invivo bioavilability studies on controlled release formulations and write the objectives and approaches in developing invitro-invivo correlation?

8. How does dissolution controlled drug delivery system differs from diffusion controlled drug delivery system?

SHORT QUESTIONS

1. Give a detail description on dissolution and diffusion controlled system.

2. Write a note on pH independent system. Note on altered density system

Chapter 2

TRANSDERMAL DRUG DELIVERY SYSTEM

2.1 INTRODUCTION

Transdermal drug delivery system has been in existence for a long time. In the past, the most commonly applied systems were topically applied creams and ointments for dermatological disorders. Today about 74% of drugs are taken orally and are found not to be as effective as desired. To improve such characters transdermal drug delivery system was emerged. Drug delivery through the skin to achieve a systemic effect of a drug is commonly known as transdermal drug delivery and differs from traditional topical drug delivery. *Transdermal drug delivery system is the system that utilizes skin as a site for continuous drug administration into the systemic circulation.* Transdermal drug delivery systems (TDDS) are dosage forms involves drug transport to viable epidermal and or dermal tissues of the skin for local therapeutic effect while a very major fraction of drug is transported into the systemic blood circulation. With the advent of new era of pharmaceutical dosage forms, transdermal drug delivery system (TDDS) established itself as an integral part of novel drug delivery systems. Transdermal drug delivery is the non-invasive delivery of medications from the surface of skin-the largest and most accessible organ of human body- through its layers, to the circulatory system. Transdermal dosage forms, though a costly alternative to conventional formulations, are becoming popular because of their unique advantages. Controlled absorption, more uniform plasma levels, improved bioavailability, reduced side effects, painless and simple application and flexibility of terminating drug administration by simply removing the patch from the skin are some of the potential advantages of transdermal drug delivery.

Transdermal drug delivery systems (TDDS), also known as "patches," are dosage forms designed to deliver a therapeutically effective amount of drug across a patient's skin. A transdermal patch or skin patch is a medicated adhesive patch that is placed on the skin to deliver a specific dose of medication through the skin and into the bloodstream. In order to deliver therapeutic agents through the human skin for systemic effects, the comprehensive morphological, biophysical and physicochemical properties of the skin are to be considered. Transdermal delivery provides a leading edge over injectables and oral routes by increasing patient compliance and avoiding first pass metabolism respectively1. Transdermal delivery not only provides controlled, constant administration of the drug, but also allows continuous input of drugs with short biological half-lives and eliminates pulsed entry into systemic circulation, which often causes undesirable side effects. FDA approved the first transdermal patch products in 1981. These delivery systems provided the controlled systemic absorption of scopolamine for the prevention of motion sickness (*Transderm-Scop*, ALZA Corp.) and Nitroglycerine for the prevention of angina pectoris associated with coronary artery disease (Transderm-Nitro).

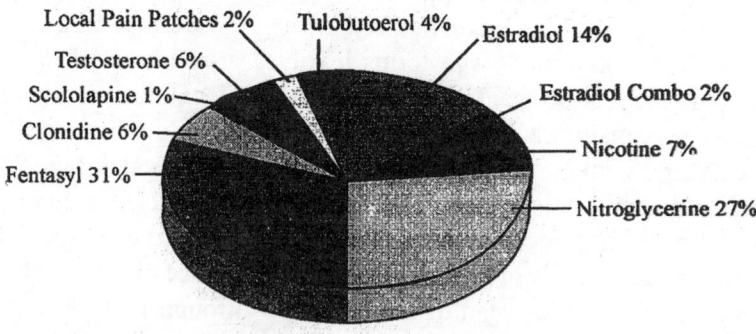

Global TDD Product Sales by Segment

Fig.1: More than 35 TDD products have now been approved for sale in the US & approximately 16 active ingredients are approved for use in TDD products globally.

2.2 OBJECTIVE OF TRANSDERMAL DRUG DELIVERY SYSTEM

➢ Delivery of the drug substance at controlled rate to intact skin of patients for absorption in to systemic circulation.

➢ System should posses proper physicochemical characteristic to permit ready release of drug substance and facilitate its partition from, delivery system in to stratum corneum.

➢ System should have a therapeutic advantage over other dosage form and drug delivery system.

➢ Patch should adhere well to patient skin and its physical size and appearance and placement on body should not be deterrent to use.

➢ The system adhesive vehicle, and active agents should be non-sensitizing nonirritating to skin of patients.

➢ System should not permit proliferation of skin bacteria beneath occlusion.

Advantages of Transdermal Drug Delivery Systems

➢ Avoids gastrointestinal tract difficulties during absorption caused by enzymes, drug interactions with food, etc.

➢ Avoids first pass i.e. the initial passage of a drug substance through the systemic and portal circulation.

➢ Provides the capacity for multi day therapy with a single application thereby improving patient compliance. Extends the activity of drugs having short half – life through the reservoir of drug present in the delivery system and its controlled release characteristics.

➢ Improved bioavailability.

➢ Reduced side effects and improved therapy due to maintenance of plasma levels up to the end of the dosing interval.

➢ Improved patient compliance and comfort via non-invasive, painless and simple application.

➢ Longer duration of action resulting in a reduction in dosing frequency.

➢ Suitable in instances like vomiting/diarrhoea where oral route is not desirable.

Disadvantages of Transdermal Drug Delivery Systems

➢ Erythema, itching, and local edema can be caused by the drug, the adhesive, or other excipients in the patch formulation.

➢ Daily dose of more than 10mg is not possible.

➢ Local irritation is a major problem.

➢ Drug requiring high blood levels are unsuitable.

➢ Drug with long half life can not be formulated in TDDS.

➢ Uncomfortable to wear.

➢ May not be economical.

➢ Barrier function changes from person to person and within the same person.

➢ Heat, cold, sweating (perspiring) and showering prevent the patch from sticking to the surface of the skin for more than one day. A new patch has to be applied daily.

Ideal Properties of Drug Candidate

For developing a transdermal drug delivery system, the drug has to be chosen with great care. Following are some Of the desirable properties of a drug suitable for transdermal delivery.

➢ The drug should have a molecular weight less than approximately 1000 Daltons.

➢ The drug should have affinity for both – lipophilic and hydrophilic phases. Extreme partitioning characteristics are not conducive to successful drug delivery via the skin.

➢ The drug should have low melting point.

➢ Along with these properties the drug should be potent, having short half life and be non irritating.

PARAMETER	PROPERTIES
Dose	Should be low (<20mg/day)
Half life	10 or less
Molecular weight	< 400
Skin permeability co- efficient	> 0.5 X 10 -3 cm/ hr
Skin reaction	Non irritating & non sensitizing
Oral Bioavailability	Low
Therapeutic index	Low

2.3 STRUCTURE OF SKIN

The skin is a multilayered Organ complex in both structure and function. Macroscopically, the skin is multilayered organ composed of many histological layers.

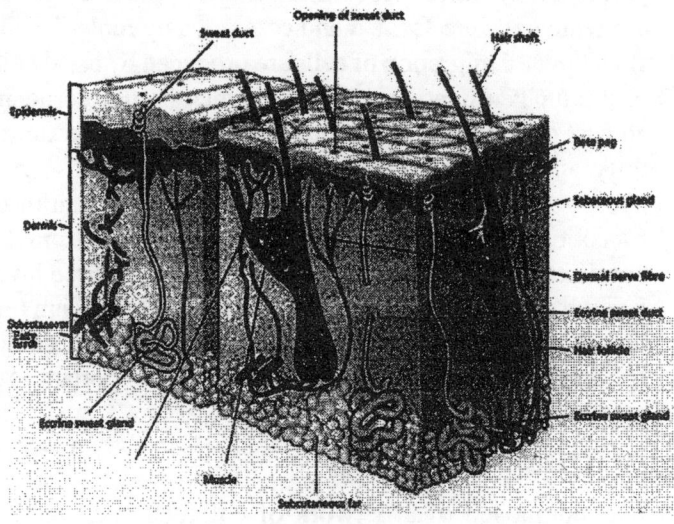

Fig.2: STRUCTURE OF SKIN

The layer of skin

1) Epidermis:

    a)   Stratum corneum (Horny cell layer)

    b)   Stratum lucidum (Clear layer)

    c)   Stratum granulosum (Granular Layer)

    d)   Stratum spinosum (Prickly layer)

    e)   Stratum germinativum

2) Dermis.

3) Hypodermis or Subcutaneous layer.

1)　EPIDERMIS

The empidermis is composed of the stratum corneum and stratum germinatum. The outermost stratum corneum layer (10-15μm thick) is quite dry and consists primarily of blocks of cytoplasmic protein matrices (keratins) embedded in extracellular lipid. The keratin containing cells, known as corneocytes, has an interlocking arrangement. Thus stratum corneum form major permeability barrier for external environment. The stratum corneum cells are formed and continuously replenished by the slow upward migration of cells are produced by basal cell layers of stratum germinativum. Most of human stratum corneum lipids consist of cermides and neutral lipids such as free sterols, free fatty acid and triglycerides. The remainder is made up of phospholipids, glycoshingolipids and cholesterol sulphate. The transition from the living cells of germinativum zone to dead, cornified cells of stratum corneum is seen in three layers: the stratum spinosum (prickly layer), stratum granulosum (granular layer) and stratum lucidem (clear layer). Stratum granulosum and stratum lucidem are also physiologically important as stratum corneum.

2)　DERMIS

It is composed of a network of collagen and elastin fibers embedded in a mucopolysaccharide matrix, which contain blood vessels, lymphatic and nerve ending thereby providing physiological support for the epidermis. It is well supplied by blood to convey nutrients, remove waste products, and regulate body temperature and pressure. Therefore the drug is well absorbed from this route.

3) SUBCUTANEOUS TISSUSE

This is a sheet of the fat containing areolar tissue known as the superficial fascia. attaching the dermis to the underlying structures.

THE SKIN APPENDAGES

ECCRINIC SWEAT GLANDS

A sweat gland produces sweat of pH 4-6.8 & absorbs drugs, secretes proteins, lipids and antibodies. Its function is to control heat.

AROCRINE SWEAT GLANDS:

It develops at pilosebcious follicle. This provides an oily secretion containing protein, lipids and lipoproteins. The surface bacteria metabolize this odourless liquid to produce the characteristic body smell.

HAIR FOLLICLES:

These develop almost all over the skin with sebaceous gland and holocrine glands to produce sebum from cell disintegration; this sebum includes glycerdes, free fatty acids, cholesterol and squalene.

2.4 MECHANISM OF ABSORPTION THROUGH SKIN

Mechanism involved is passive diffusion

This can be expressed by FICK's LAW of DIFFUSION

$$dq/dt = D K A (c_1 - c_2)/h$$

$dq/dt =$ rate of diffusion

D = diffusion co-efficient

K = partition co- efficient

A = surface area of membrane

H = thickness of membrane.

There are two potential route of absorption:

1) Hair follicular/ sweat gland (Transfollicular route).

2) Stratum corneum (Transepidermal route).

1).TRANSFOLLICULAR ROUTE

Fractional area available through this route is 0.1 %. Human skin contains 40-70 hair follicles, 200 to 250 sweat glands on every sq.cm. Of skin area.

Mainly water soluble substance is diffused faster through appendages than that of other layers. Sweat glands and hair follicles act as a shunt i.e. easy pathway for diffusion through rate limiting stratum corneum.

2). TRANSEPIDERMAL ROUTE

Epidermal barrier function mainly resides in horny layer. The viable layer may metabolize, inactivate or activate a prodrug. Dermal capillary contains many capillaries so residence time of drug is only one minute. Within stratum corneum molecule may penetrate either transcellularly or intercellularly. Intracellular region is filled with lipid rich amorphous material.

There are two possible ways of diffusion:

a) Transcellular – diffusion occur through the cells.

b) Interacellular – diffusion occur through the intercellular space present between the cells.

For the water soluble, non electrolytes are not primarily by intercellular. Transcellular permeation is explained on the basis of relatively samller diffusion coefficient. Thus molecular diffusion through interacellular, can also penetrate through transcelluar. The viable epidermis is considered as single field of diffusion. It is permeable field that function at hydrolhillic extremes but for lipophilic and electrolytes functions as hydrophobic extremes which have difficulty in passing through viable field. The viable tissue is rate determining when non polar compounds are invaded.

2.5 TYPES OF TRANSDERMAL DELIVERY SYSTEMS

All Transdermal drug delivery system have a basic structure comprising of many layers, having specific function.

➤ Backing layer: Preventing wetting of system during use.

➤ Reservoir layer: supplies continuous quantum of drug for predetermined functional life time of system.

➤ Rate control polymeric membrane: Regulates the rate of drug during a predetermined time interval.

Rate of drug release from the transdermal drug delivery system is normally much greater than amount that the skin can absorb. Hence even if there is variation in skin permeability, a constant rate of drug input into circulation is achieved.

Preparation of Different Types of Transdermal Patches

➤ MEMBRANE MODERATED TRANSDERMAL DRUG DELIVERY SYSTEM.

➤ ADHESIVE DIFFUSION CONTROLLED TRANSDERMAL DRUG DELIVERY SYSTEM.

➤ MATRIX DISPERSION TRANSDERMAL DRUG DELIVERY SYSTEM.

➤ MICRO RESERVOIR TRANSDERMAL DRUG DELIVERY SYSTEM.

A) MEMBRANE MODERATED TRANSDERMAL DRUG DELIVERY SYSTEM

In this membrane moderated approach the drug reservoir is encapsulated in a shallow compartment moulded from a drug impermeable metallic-plastic lamination while the drug delivery side is covered by rate controlling polymeric membrane. In the drug reservoir compartment the drug solid matrix is suspended in unleachable viscous fluid that forms paste like suspension.

On the external surface, a thin layer of drug compatible adhesive polymer may be applied for an intimate delivery phase to skin contact. The rate of drug release from this type of transdermal drug delivery system can be tailored by varying the polymer composition, permeability coefficient and thickness of the rate controlling membrane.

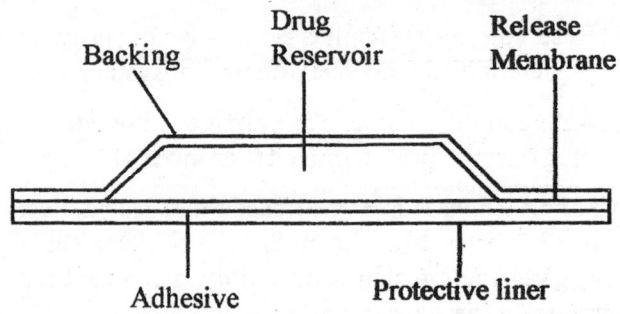

Fig.3: MEMBRANE MODERATED TRANSDERMAL DRUG DELIVERY SYSTEM

Eg. TransdermScop – for 3day medication of motion sickness.

TransdermNitro – for once a day medication of angina pectoris.

This approach has also been used for development of tarnsdermal therapeutic system for controlled percutaneous absorption of estradiol, clonidine and prostaglandin.

B) ADHESIVE DIFFUSION CONTROLLED TRANSDERMAL DRUG DELIVERY SYSTEM

This type of delivery system is a simplified form of membrane moderated drug delivery system; instead of completely encapsulating the drug reservoir in a compartment, the drug reservoir is prepared by direct dispensing the drug in an adhesive polymer and then spreading the medicated adhesive by solvent film casting method over a flat sheet of drug impermeable metallic/plastic backing membrane. This forms a thin drug reservoir layer. The drug reservoir later is then covered by non-diffusion controlling drug delivery system.

Eg: Deponit system/ pharma-Schwartz Nitroglycerin once a day in angina pectoris. Frandol tape/ Toaeiyo Nitroglycerin Once a day in angina pectoris. This system is also applied for controlled administration of verapamil.

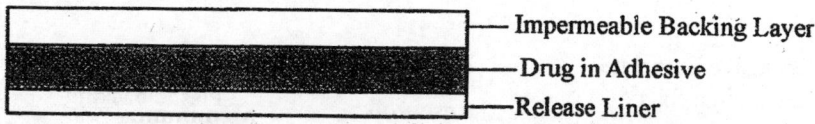

— Impermeable Backing Layer
— Drug in Adhesive
— Release Liner

Fig.4: ADHESIVE DIFFUSION CONTROLLED TRANSDERMAL DRUG DELIVERY SYSTEM

C) MATRIX DIFFUSION TRANSDERMAL DRUG DELIVERY SYSTEM.

Drug reservoir is prepared by dissolving the drug and polymer in a common solvent. The insoluble drug should be homogenously dispersed in hydrophilic or lipophillic polymer. The required quantity of plasticizer like dibutylpthalate, triethylcitrate, polyethylene glycol or propylene glycol and permeation enhancer is then added and mixed properly. The medicated polymer formed is then molded into rings with defined surface area and controlled thickness over the mercury on horizontal surface followed by solvent evaporation at an elevated temperature. The film formed is then separated from the rings, which is then mounted onto an occlusive base plate in a compartment fabricated from a drug impermeable backing. Adhesive polymer is then spread along the circumference of the film. Commonly used polymers for matrix are cross linked polyethylene glycol, eudragits, ethyl cellulose, polyvinylpyrrolidone and hydroxypropylmethylcellulose.

The dispersion of drug particles in the polymer matrix can be accomplished by either homogenously mixing the finely ground drug particles with a liquid polymer or a highly viscous base polymer followed by cross linking of polymer chains or homogenously blending drug solids with a rubbery polymer at an elevated temperature.

Eg: Nitro-dur/ key Nitroglycerin once a day in angina pectoris.

Estradiol diacetate.

Verapamil.

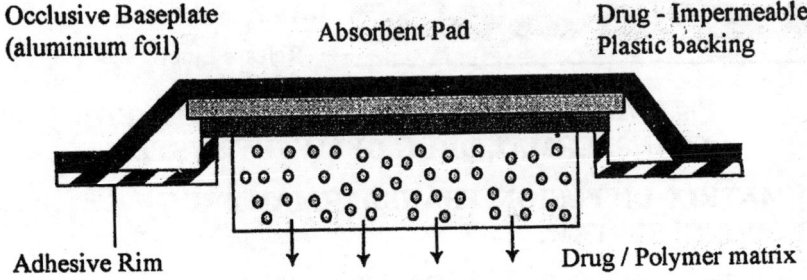

Occlusive Baseplate (aluminium foil)   Absorbent Pad   Drug - Impermeable Plastic backing

Adhesive Rim   Drug / Polymer matrix

Fig.5: MATRIX DIFFUSION TRANSDERMAL DRUG DELIVERY SYSTEM.

D) MICRO RESERVOIR TRANSDERMAL DRUG DELIVERY SYSTEM.

In this type the drug delivery system is a combination of reservoir and matrix-dispersion system. The drug reservoir is formed by first suspending the drug in an aqueous solution of water soluble polymer and then dispersing the solution homogeneously in a lipophilic polymer to form thousands of unreachable, microscopic spheres of drug reservoirs. This thermodynamically unstable dispersion is stabilized quickly by immediately cross-linking the polymer in situ by using cross linking agents. A transdermal therapeutic system thus formed as a medicated disc positioned at centre and surrounded by an adhesive rim.

Eg. Nitro-dur/ seale for once day treatment of angina pectoris.

Microscopic

Drug Reservoir

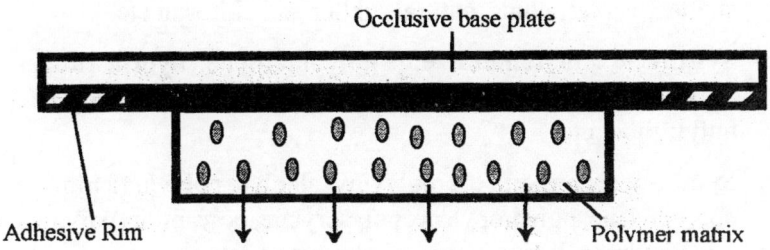

Fig.6: MICRO RESERVOIR TRANSDERMAL DRUG DELIVERY SYSTEM.

2.6 BASIC COMPONENTS USED FOR TRANSDERMAL DRUG DELIVERY SYSTEM

➢ Polymer matrix.

➢ Drug.

➢ Permeation enhancers.

➢ Other excipients – Adhesive and Backing membrane.

1) POLYMER MATRIX

Polymers are the backbone of TDDS, which control the release of the drug from the device. Polymer matrix can be prepared by dispersion of drug in liquid or solid state synthetic polymer base. Polymers used in TDDS should have biocompatibility and chemical compatibility with the drug and other components of the system such as penetration enhancers and Pressure sensitive adhesive (PSAs). Additionally they should provide consistent and effective delivery of a drug throughout the product's intended shelf life and should be of safe status.

THE POLYMERS UTILIZED FOR TDDS CAN BE CLASSIFIED AS

- ➢ **Natural Polymers:** e.g. cellulose derivatives, zein, gelatin, shellac, waxes, gums, natural rubber and chitosan etc.

- ➢ **Synthetic Elastomers:** e.g. polybutadiene, hydrin rubber, polyisobutylene, silicon rubber, nitrile, acrylonitrile, neoprene, butylrubber etc.

- ➢ **Synthetic Polymers:** e.g. polyvinyl alcohol, polyvinylchloride, polyethylene, polypropylene, polyacrylate, polyamide, polyurea, polyvinylpyrrolidone, polymethylmethacrylate etc.

The polymers like cross linked polyethylene glycol, eudragits, ethyl cellulose, polyvinylpyrrolidone and hydroxypropylmethylcellulose are used as matrix formers for TDDS. Other polymers like ethylene vinyl acetate (EVA), silicon rubber and polyurethane are used as rate controlling membrane.

The Polymer Should Fulfill The Following Requirements:

- ➢ Molecular weight, physical characteristics and chemical funtionalitity of the polymer must allow the diffusion of the drug substances at desirable rate.

- ➢ The polymer should be chemically non reactive or it should be inert drug carrier.

- ➢ The polymer must not decompose on storage or during the life of device.

- ➢ The polymer and its decomposed product should be nontoxic.

- ➢ The polymer must be easy to manufacture and fabricate into the desired product.

- ➢ Mechanical properties of polymer should not deteriorate excessively where large amount of active agent are incorporated into in.

- ➢ The cost of the polymer should not be excessively high or inexpensive.

2) DRUG

The transdermal route is an extremely attractive option for the drugs with appropriate pharmacology and physical chemistry. Transdermal patches offer much to drugs which undergo extensive first pass metabolism, drugs with narrow therapeutic window, or drugs with short half life which causes non- compliance due to frequent dosing. The foremost requirement of TDDS is that the drug possesses the right mix of physicochemical and biological properties for transdermal drug delivery. It is generally accepted that the best drug candidates for passive adhesive transdermal patches must be non ionic, of low molecular weight (less than 500 Daltons), have adequate solubility in oil and water (log P in the range of 1-3), a low melting point (less than 200°C) and are potent (dose in mg per day).

Eg: Nicotine, Methotrexate and Estrogen.

3) PERMEATION ENHANCERS

Permeation enhancers controls the release of the drug. These are the promotes skin permeability by altering the skin as a barrier of flux of desired penetrant. They are the chemical compounds that increase permeability of stratum corneum so as to attain higher therapeutic levels of the drug candidate. Penetration enhancers interact with structural components of stratum corneum i.e., proteins or lipids. They alter the protein and lipid packaging of stratum corneum, thus chemically modifying the barrier functions leading to increased permeability.

Ex: Terpenes, Terpenoids, Pyrrolidones. Solvents like alcohol, Ethanol, Methanol. Surfactants like Sodium Lauryl sulfate, Pluronic F127, Pluronic F68.

CHARACTERISTICS OF PERMEATION ENHANCERS

Permeation enhancer should be:

➢ Pharmacologically inert.

➢ Nontoxic, nonirritating and non allergic.

➢ Immediate action and should be suitable and predictable action.

➤ Upon removal, skin should be immediately and fully recover its normal barrier properties.

➤ Compatible with all drug and exicipents.

➤ Odourless, elastic, colorless and inexpensive.

MECHANISM OF PREMEATION ENHANCER

They act by three mechanisms:

1) Reduces the resistance of stratum corneum by altering its physicochemical properties.

2) Alteration of hydration of stratum corneum.

3) Affecting the structure of lipids and protein in intercellular channel through solvent action or denaturation and also sometime the carrier mechanism is observed.

4) Other excipients

a) Adhesives: Serves to adhere the patch to the skin for systemic delivery of drug. Adhesive is a material that helps in maintaining an intimate contact between transdermal system and the skin surface. It should adhere with not more than applied finger pressure, be aggressively and permanently tachy, exert a strong holding force. Additionally, it should be removable from the smooth surface without leaving a residue. Polyacrylates, polyisobutylene and silicon based adhesives are widely used in TDDSs. The selection of an adhesive is based on numerous factors, including the patch design and drug formulation. Ideally, Adhesive should be physicochemically and biologically compatible and should not alter drug release. Should not irritate or sensitize skin or cause imbalance in normal skin flora during its contact time with skin. Pressure sensitive adhesive are generally used e.g polysobutylenes, acrylic and silicons.

b) Backing membrane: They protect patch from outer environment. While designing a backing layer, the consideration of chemical resistance of the material is most important. Excipient compatibility should also be considered because the prolonged contact between the backing layer and the excipients may cause the additives to leach out of the backing layer or may lead to diffusion of excipients, drug or penetration enhancer through the layer. However, an overemphasis on the chemical resistance may lead to stiffness and high occlusivity to moisture vapor and air, causing patches to lift and possibly irritate the skin during long wear. The most comfortable backing will be the one that exhibits lowest modulus or high flexibility, good oxygen transmission and a high moisture vapor transmission rate.

Examples of some backing materials are vinyl, polyethylene, polyester films, Cellulose derivatives, poly vinyl alcohol, and Polypropylene Silicon rubber.

Evaluation of Transdermal Patches

Development of controlled release transdermal dosage form is a complex process involving extensive research. Transdermal patches have been developed to improve clinical efficacy of the drug and to enhance patient compliance by delivering smaller amount of drug at a predetermined rate. This makes evaluation studies even more important in order to ensure their desired performance and reproducibility under the specified environmental conditions. These studies are predictive of transdermal dosage forms and can be classified into following types:

- Physicochemical evaluation.
- In vitro evaluation.
- In vivo evaluation.

a) Physicochemical evaluation

1. **Thickness:** The thickness of the drug loaded patch is measured in different points by using a digital micrometer, traveling microscope, dial gauge, screw gauge. And determines the average thickness and standard deviation for the same to ensure the thickness of the prepared patch.

2. **Uniformity of weight:** Weight variation is studied by individually weighing 10 randomly selected patches. A specified area of patch is to be cut in different parts of the patch and weigh in digital balance. The average weight and standard deviation values are to be calculated from the individual weights.

3.   **Drug content determination:** An accurately weighed portion of film (about 100 mg) is dissolved in 100 ml of suitable solvent in which drug is soluble and then the solution is shaken continuously for 24 hrs in shaker incubator. Then the whole solution is sonicated. After sonication and subsequent filtration, drug in solution is estimated spectrophotometrically by appropriate dilution.

4.   **Content uniformity test:** 10 patches are selected and content is determined for individual patches. If 9 out of 10 patches have content between 85% to 115% of the specified value and one has content not less than 75% to 125% of the specified value, then transdermal patches pass the test of content uniformity. But if 3 patches have content in the range of 75% to 125%, then additional 20 patches are tested for drug content. If these 20 patches have range from 85% to 115%, then the transdermal patches pass the test.

5.   **Percentage Moisture content:** The weighed films are to be kept in a desiccator at room temperature for 24 hrs containing saturated solution of potassium chloride in order to maintain 84% RH. After 24 hrs the films are to be reweighed and determine the percentage moisture uptake from the below mentioned formula.

Moisture content = [Initial weight- Final weight/ Final weight] × 100.

6.   **Percentage Moisture Uptake:**

The weighed films are to be kept in a desiccator at room temperature for 24 hrs containing saturated solution of potassium chloride in order to maintain 84% RH. After 24 hrs the films are to be reweighed and determine the percentage moisture uptake from the below mentioned formula.

Percentage moisture uptake = [Final weight- Initial weight/ initial weight] × 100.

7.   **Water vapor permeability (WVP) evaluation:**

Water vapor permeability can be determined with foam dressing method the air forced oven is replaced by a natural air circulation oven. The WVP can be determined by the following formula

$$WVP=W/A$$

Where, WVP is expressed in gm/m2 per 24hrs,

W is the amount of vapor permeated through the patch expressed in gm/24hrs and,

A is the surface area of the exposure samples expressed in m.

8. **Folding Endurance:** Evaluation of folding endurance involves determining the folding capacity of the films subjected to frequent extreme conditions of folding. Folding endurance is determined by repeatedly folding the film at the same place until it break. The number of times the films could be folded at the same place without breaking is folding endurance value.

9. **Tensile Strength:** The tensile strength should be determined by using a modified pulley system. Weight was gradually increased so as to increase the pulling force till the patch broke. The force required to break the film was consider as a tensile strength and it was calculated as kg/cm^2.

10. **Flatness:** Three longitudinal strips should be cut out from each film: one from the center, one from the left side, and one from the right side. The length of each strip should be measured and the variation in length because of non-uniformity in flatness was measured by determining percent constriction, is 0% constriction equivalent to 100% flatness.

Adhesive studies

The therapeutic performance of TDDS can be affected by the quality of contact between the patch and the skin. The adhesion of a TDDS to the skin is obtained by using pressure sensitive adhesives (PSAs), which are defined as adhesives capable of bonding to surfaces with the application of light pressure. The adhesive properties of a TDDS can be characterized by considering the following factors:

Peel Adhesion test

In this test, the force required to remove an adhesive coating form a test substrate is referred to as peel adhesion. Molecular weight of adhesive polymer, the type and amount of additives are the variables that determined the peel adhesion properties. A single tape is applied to a stainless steel plate or a backing membrane of choice and then tape is pulled from the substrate at a 180° angle, and the force required for tape removed is measured.

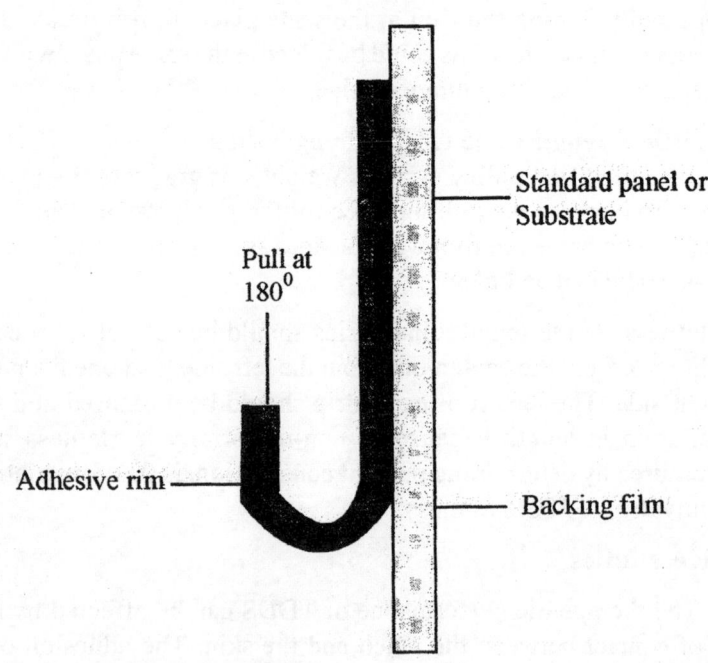

Fig.7: Peel Adhesion test.

Tack properties: It is the ability of the polymer to adhere to substrate with little contact pressure. Tack is dependent on molecular weight and composition of polymer as well as on the use of tackifying resins in polymer.

Thumb tack test: The force required to remove thumb from adhesive is a measure of tack. It is a qualitative test applied for tack property determination of adhesive. The thumb is simply pressed on the adhesive and the relative tack property is detected.

Rolling ball test: This test involves measurement of the distance that stainless steel ball travels along an upward facing adhesive. In this the, stainless steel ball of 7/16 inches in diameter is released on an inclined track so that it rolls down and comes into contact with horizontal, upward facing adhesive. The distance the ball travels along the adhesive provides the measurement of tack, which is expressed in inch. The less tacky the adhesive, the further the ball will travel.

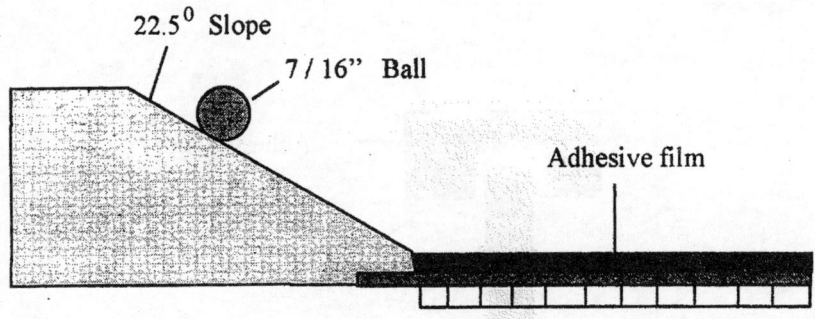

Fig.8: Rolling ball test.

Quick Stick (peel-tack) test: In this test, the tape is pulled away from the substrate at 90°C at a speed of 12 inches/min. The peel force required breaking the bond between adhesive and substrate is measured and recorded as tack value, which is expressed in ounces or grams per inch width.

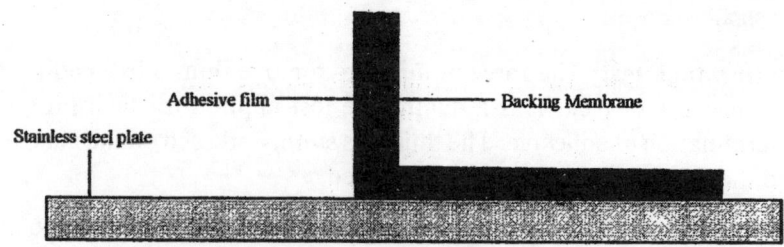

Fig.9: Quick stick test for adhesive evaluation.

Probe Tack test: In this test, the tip of a clean probe with a defined surface roughness is brought into contact with adhesive, and when a bond is formed between probe and adhesive. The subsequent removal of the probe mechanically breaks it. The force required to pull the probe away from the adhesive at fixed rate is recorded as tack and it is expressed in grams.

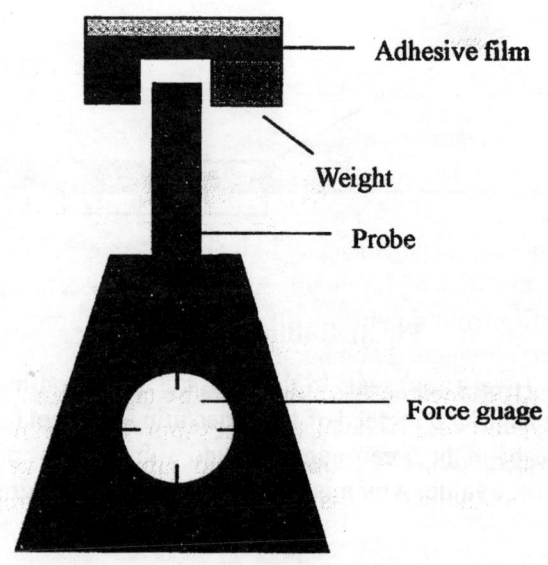

Fig.10: Probe Tack test.

Shear strength properties or creep resistance: Shear strength is the measurement of the cohesive strength of an adhesive polymer i.e., device should not slip on application determined by measuring the time it takes to pull an adhesive coated tape off a stainless plate.

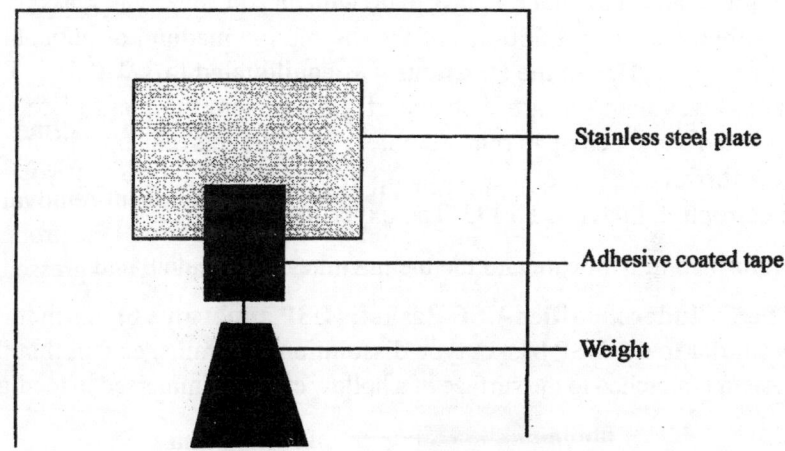

Stainless steel plate

Adhesive coated tape

Weight

Fig.11: Shear strength properties or creep resistance

In vitro release studies

Drug release mechanisms and kinetics are two characteristics of the dosage forms which play an important role in describing the drug dissolution profile from a controlled release dosage forms and hence there in vivo performance. A number of mathematical model have been developed to describe the drug dissolution kinetics from controlled release drug delivery system e.g., Higuchi, First order, Zero order and Peppas and Korsenmeyer model. The dissolution data is fitted to these models and the best fit is obtained to describe the release mechanism of the drug.

There are various methods available for determination of drug release rate of TDDS.

The Paddle over Disc: (USP apparatus 5)

The paddle over disc method (USP apparatus V) can be employed for assessment of the release of the drug from the prepared patches. Dry films of known thickness is to be cut into definite shape, weighed, and fixed over a glass plate with an adhesive. The glass plate was then placed in a 500-mL of the dissolution medium or phosphate buffer (pH 7.4), and the apparatus was equilibrated to 32± 0.5°C. The paddle was then set at a distance of 2.5 cm from the glass plate and operated at a speed of 50 rpm. Samples (5-ml aliquots) can be withdrawn at appropriate time intervals up to 24 h and analyzed by UV spectrophotometer or HPLC. The experiment is to be performed in triplicate and the mean value can be calculated.

The Cylinder modified USP Basket: (USP apparatus 6) this method is similar to the USP basket type dissolution apparatus, except that the system is attached to the surface of a hollow cylinder immersed in medium at 32 ±5°.

The reciprocating disc: (USP apparatus 7): In this method patches attached to holders are oscillated in small volumes of medium, allowing the apparatus to be useful for systems delivering low concentration of drug. In addition paddle over extraction cell method may be used.

Diffusion Cells e.g. Franz Diffusion Cell and its modification Keshary- Chien Cell

In this method transdermal system is placed in between receptor and donor compartment of the diffusion cell. The transdermal system faces the receptor compartment in which receptor fluid i.e., buffer is placed. The agitation speed and temperature are kept constant. The whole assembly is kept on magnetic stirrer and solution in the receiver compartment is constantly and continuously stirred throughout the experiment using magnetic beads. At predetermined time intervals, the receptor fluid is removed for analysis and is replaced with an equal volume of fresh receptor fluid. The concentration of drug is determined spectrophotometrically.

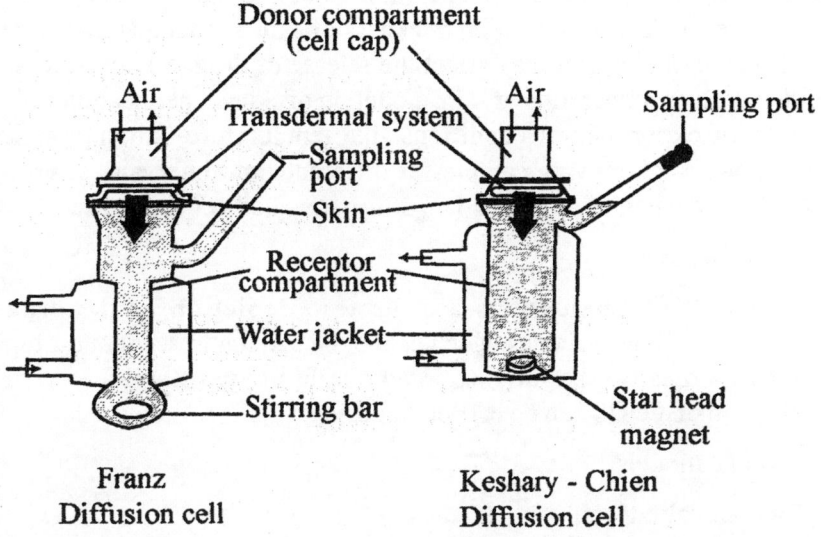

Fig.12: Diffusion Cells

In vitro permeation studies

The amount of drug available for absorption to the systemic pool is greatly dependent on drug released from the polymeric transdermal films. The drug reached at skin surface is then passed to the dermal microcirculation by penetration through cells of epidermis, between the cells of epidermis through skin appendages. Usually permeation studies are performed by placing the fabricated transdermal patch with rat skin or synthetic membrane in between receptor and donor compartment in a vertical diffusion cell such as franz diffusion cell or keshary-chien diffusion cell. The transdermal system is applied to the hydrophilic side of the membrane and then mounted in the diffusion cell with lipophillic side in contact with receptor fluid. The receiver compartment is maintained at specific temperature (usually 32±5°C for skin) and is continuously stirred at a constant rate. The samples are withdrawn at different time intervals and equal amount of buffer is replaced each time. The samples are diluted appropriately and absorbance is determined spectrophotometrically. Then the amount of drug permeated per centimeter square at each time interval is calculated. Design of system, patch size, surface area of skin, thickness of skin and temperature etc. are some variables that may affect the release of drug. So permeation study involves preparation of skin, mounting of skin on permeation cell, setting of experimental conditions like temperature, stirring, sink conditions, withdrawing samples at different time intervals, sample analysis and calculation of flux i.e., drug permeated per cm^2 per second.

In vivo Studies

In vivo evaluations are the true depiction of the drug performance. The variables which cannot be taken into account during in vitro studies can be fully explored during in vivo studies. In vivo evaluation of TDDS can be carried out using:

a). Animal models

b).Human volunteers.

Animal models

Considerable time and resources are required to carry out human studies, so animal studies are preferred at small scale. The most common animal species used for evaluating transdermal drug delivery system are mouse, hairless rat, hairless dog, hairless rhesus monkey, rabbit, guinea pig etc. Various experiments conducted lead us to a conclusion that hairless animals are preferred over hairy animals in both in vitro and in vivo experiments. Rhesus monkey is one of the most reliable models for in vivo evaluation of transdermal drug delivery in man.

Human models

The final stage of the development of a transdermal device involves collection of pharmacokinetic and pharmacodynamic data following application of the patch to human volunteers. Clinical trials have been conducted to assess the efficacy, risk involved, side effects, patient compliance etc. Phase I clinical trials are conducted to determine mainly safety in volunteers and phase II clinical trials determine short term safety and mainly effectiveness in patients. Phase III trials indicate the safety and effectiveness in large number of patient population and phase IV trials at post marketing surveillance are done for marketed patches to detect adverse drug reactions. Though human studies require considerable resources but they are the best to assess the performance of the drug.

REVIEW QUESTIONS

ESSAY QUESTIONS

1. What criteria are necessary for a drug to be given by Transdermal Drug Delivery Systems and write the mechanisam of transdermal permeation?

2. Which components are required for the design of Transdermal Drug Delivery Systems?

3. What are various approaches for the developement of TDDS?

4. Which factors are considered in selecting an invitro skin Permeation studies and write about description of Franz diffusion cell?

5. Write Advantages and Disadvantages of Transdermal Drug Delivery Systems and formula for Water vapour transmission, Permeability Co efficient and Diffusion flux?

6. Write about description of In-Vitro Dissolution study Apparatus for TDDS and write Acceptancy criteria as per USP?

7. What are In-vivo Evaluation techniques for Transdermal Drug Delivery Systems and Write In-vivo Evaluation procedure by taking any one animal model?

8. Write about Sample size, Exclusion Criteria, Duration of Study, Study Design and Data presentation of Skin irritation study and Skin Sensitization study?

SHORT QUESTIONS

1. Brief out the mechanism involved in drug absorption through skin.

2. Give the ideal drug characteristics for transdermal drug delivery system and mention the advantages and disadvantages of TDDS.

3. Write a note on permeation enhancers and give its mechanism

Chapter 3

MUCOADHESIVE DELIVERY SYSTEMS

3.1 INTRODUCTION

Oral drug delivery has been known for decades as the most widely utilized route of administration among all the routes that have been explored for the systemic delivery of drugs via various pharmaceutical products of different dosage forms. The reasons that the oral route achieved such popularity may be in part attributed to its ease of administration as well as the traditional belief that by oral administration the drug is well absorbed as the food stuffs that are ingested daily. In 1986, Longer and Robinson defined the term bioadhesion as the attachment of a synthetic or natural macromolecule to mucus and/or an epithelial surface Mucoadhesion is a topic of current interest in the design of drug delivery systems. Mucoadhesive drug delivery system prolong the residence time of the dosage form at the site of application or absorption and facilitate an intimate contact of the dosage form with the underline absorption surface and thus contribute to improved and / or better therapeutic performance of the drug. In recent years many such mucoadhesive drug delivery systems have been developed for oral, buccal, nasal, rectal and vaginal routes for both systemic and local effects.

Bioadhesion can be defined as a phenomenon of interfacial molecular attractive forces amongst the surfaces of the biological substrate and the natural or synthetic polymers, which allows the polymer to adhere to the biological surface for an extended period of time. When the biological substrate is a mucosal layer then the phenomena is known as mucoadhesion. Bioadhesive polymeric systems have been used since long time in the development of products for various biomedical applications which include denture adhesives and surgical glue. The adhesion of bacteria to the human gut may be attributed to the interaction of lectin-like structure (present on the cell surface of bacteria) and mucin (present in the biological tissues). In general, various biopolymers show the bioadhesive properties and have been utilized for various therapeutic purposes in medicine. Mucoadhesive polymers as drug delivery vehicles. The common principle underlying this drug administration route is the adhesion of the dosage form to the mucous layer until the polymer dissolves or the mucin replaces itself. Benefits for this route of drug administration are: prolonged drug delivery, targeted therapy and often improved bioavailability. Bioadhesion is the state in which two materials, (at least one of which is biological in nature), are held together for a extended period of time by interfacial forces. The term bioadhesion implies attachment of drug-carrier system to specific biological location. This biological surface can be epithelial tissue or the mucous coat on the surface of tissue.

Within the oral mucosal cavity, delivery of drugs is classified into three categories.

1) **Sublingual delivery**: which is systemic delivery of drugs through the mucosal membranes lining the floor of the mouth.

2) **Buccal delivery**: which is drug administration through the mucosal membranes lining the cheeks (buccal mucosa), and

3) **Local delivery**: which is drug delivery into the oral cavity

Concepts

In biological systems, four types of bioadhesion could be distinguished:

1. Adhesion of a normal cell on another normal cell.

2. Adhesion of a cell with a foreign substance.

3. Adhesion of a normal cell to a pathological cell.

4. .Adhesion of an adhesive to a biological substance.

For drug delivery purpose, the term bioadhesion implies attachment of a drug carrier system to a specific biological location. The biological surface can be epithelial tissue. If adhesive attachment is to a mucus coat, the phenomenon is referred to as mucoadhesion. Bioadhesion can be modeled after a bacterial attachment to tissue surfaces, and mucoadhesion can be modeled after the adherance of mucus on epithelial tissue.

Advantages

➤ It is richly vascularized and more accessible for the administration and removal of a dosage form.

➤ Termination of therapy is possible.

➤ Permits localization of drug to the oral cavity for extended period of time.

➤ Ease of administration.

➤ Avoids acid hydrolysis in the gastrointestinal (GI) tract and by passing the first-pass effect.

➤ Reduction in dose can be achieved, thereby reducing dose dependent side effects.

➤ It allows local modification of tissue permeability, inhibition of protease activity or reduction in immunogenic response, thus selective use of therapeutic agents like peptides, proteins and ionized species can be achieved.

➤ Drugs which are unstable in acidic environment of stomach or destroyed by the alkaline environment of intestine can be given by this route.

➤ Drugs which show poor bioavailability by oral route can be administered by this route.

➤ Drugs with short half life can be administered by this method. (2-8 hrs)

e.g. :- nitroglycerin (2 hrs) isosorbide mononitrate (2-5 hrs).

Disadvantages

➢ Over hydration may lead to formation of slippery surface & structural integrity of the formulation may get disrupted by the swelling & hydration of the bioadhesive polymer.

➢ Eating and drinking may become restricted.

➢ There is possibility that Patient may swallow the tablet.

➢ The drug contained in swallowed saliva follows the per oral route & advantages of buccal route is lost.

➢ Only drug with small dose requirement can be administered.

➢ Drug which irritate mucosa or have a bitter or unpleasant taste or an obnoxious odour cannot be administered by this route.

➢ Drugs which are unstable at buccal pH cannot be administered by this route.

➢ Only those drugs which are absorbed by passive diffusion can be administered by this route.

Ideal Candidates For Buccal Drug Delivery Systems

➢ Molecular size 75 – 100 Daltons, Molecular weight 200 – 500 Daltons.

➢ Drugs should be preferably lipophilic in nature (for transcellular absorption).

➢ Drug should be odorless.

➢ Drugs which are absorbed only by passive diffusion should be used.

➢ Drug should be stable at buccal pH (6.4 – 7.2)g.

3.2 OVERVIEW OF THE ORAL MUCOSA

A. Structure

The oral mucosa is composed of an outermost layer of stratified squamous epithelium (Figure 1). Below this lies a basement membrane, a lamina propria followed by the submucosa as the innermost layer. The epithelium is similar to stratified squamous epithelia found in the rest of the body in that it has a mitotically active basal cell layer, advancing through a number of differentiating intermediate layers to the superficial layers, where cells are shed from the surface of the epithelium. The epithelium of the buccal mucosa is about 40-50 cell layers thick, while that of the sublingual epithelium contains somewhat fewer. The epithelial cells increase in size and become flatter as they travel from the basal layers to the superficial layers.

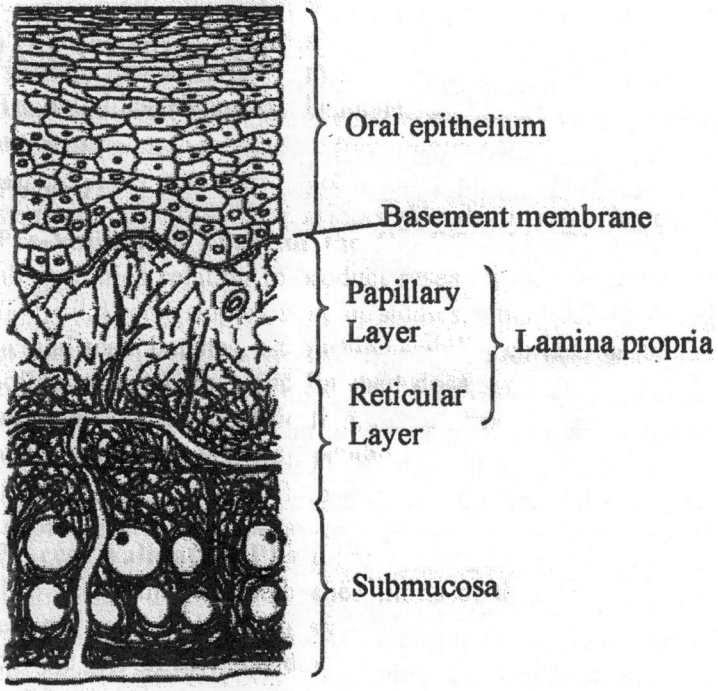

Oral epithelium

Basement membrane

Papillary Layer

Reticular Layer

Lamina propria

Submucosa

Fig.1: Structure of the oral mucosa.

The turnover time for the buccal epithelium has been estimated at 5-6 days, and this is probably representative of the oral mucosa as a whole. The oral mucosal thickness varies depending on the site: the buccal mucosa measures at 500-800 µm, while the mucosal thickness of the hard and soft palates, the floor of the mouth, the ventral tongue, and the gingivae measure at about 100-200 µm. The composition of the epithelium also varies depending on the site in the oral cavity. The mucosae of areas subject to mechanical stress (the gingivae and hard palate) are keratinized similar to the epidermis. The mucosae of the soft palate, the sublingual, and the buccal regions, however, are not keratinized. The keratinized epithelia contain neutral lipids like ceramides and acylceramides which have been associated with the barrier function. These epithelia are relatively impermeable to water. In contrast, non-keratinized epithelia, such as the floor of the mouth and the buccal epithelia, do not contain acylceramides and only have small amounts of ceramide. They also contain small amounts of neutral but polar lipids, mainly cholesterol sulfate and glucosyl ceramides. These epithelia have been found to be considerably more permeable to water than keratinized epithelia.

B. Permeability

The oral mucosae in general is a somewhat leaky epithelia intermediate between that of the epidermis and intestinal mucosa. It is estimated that the permeability of the buccal mucosa is 4-4000 times greater than that of the skin. As indicative by the wide range in this reported value, there are considerable differences in permeability between different regions of the oral cavity because of the diverse structures and functions of the different oral mucosae. In general, the permeabilities of the oral mucosae decrease in the order of sublingual greater than buccal, and buccal greater than palatal. This rank order is based on the relative thickness and degree of keratinization of these tissues, with the sublingual mucosa being relatively thin and non-keratinized, the buccal thicker and non-keratinized, and the palatal intermediate in thickness but keratinized. It is currently believed that the permeability barrier in the oral mucosa is a result of intercellular material derived from the so-called 'membrane coating granules' (MCG). When cells go through differentiation, MCGs start forming and at the apical cell surfaces they fuse with the plasma membrane and their contents are discharged into the intercellular spaces at the upper one third of the epithelium. This barrier exists in the outermost 200µm of the superficial layer. Permeation studies have been performed using a number of very large molecular weight tracers, such as horseradish peroxidase and lanthanum nitrate. When applied to the outer surface of the epithelium, these tracers penetrate only through outermost layer or two of cells. When applied to the submucosal surface, they permeate up to, but not into, the outermost cell layers of the epithelium. According to these results, it seems apparent that flattened surface cell layers present the main barrier to permeation, while the more isodiametric cell layers are relatively permeable. In both keratinized and non-keratinized epithelia, the limit of penetration coincided with the level where the MCGs could be seen adjacent to the superficial plasma membranes of the epithelial cells. Since the same result was obtained in both keratinized and non-keratinized epithelia, keratinization by itself is not expected to play a significant role in the barrier function . The components of the MCGs in keratinized and non-keratinized epithelia are different, however. The MCGs of keratinized epithelium are composed of lamellar lipid stacks, whereas the non-keratinized epithelium contains MCGs that are non-lamellar. The MCG lipids of keratinized epithelia include sphingomyelin, glucosylceramides, ceramides, and other nonpolar lipids, however for non-keratinized epithelia, the major MCG lipid components are cholesterol esters, cholesterol, and glycosphingolipids. Aside from the MCGs, the basement membrane may present some resistance to permeation as well, however the outer epithelium is still considered to be the rate limiting step to mucosal penetration. The structure of the basement membrane is not dense enough to exclude even relatively large molecules.

C. Environment

The cells of the oral epithelia are surrounded by an intercellular ground substance, mucus, the principle components of which are complexes made up of proteins and carbohydrates. These complexes may be free of association or some maybe attached to certain regions on the cell surfaces. This matrix may actually play a role in cell-cell adhesion, as well as acting as a lubricant, allowing cells to move relative to one another. Along the same lines, the mucus is also believed to play a role in bioadhesion of mucoadhesive drug delivery systems. In stratified squamous epithelia found elsewhere in the body, mucus is synthesized by specialized mucus secreting cells like the goblet cells, however in the oral mucosa, mucus is secreted by the major and minor salivary glands as part of saliva. Up to 70% of the total mucin found in saliva is contributed by the minor salivary glands. At physiological pH the mucus network carries a negative charge (due to the sialic acid and sulfate residues) which may play a role in mucoadhesion. At this pH mucus can form a strongly cohesive gel structure that will bind to the epithelial cell surface as a gelatinous layer. Another feature of the environment of the oral cavity is the presence of saliva produced by the salivary glands. Saliva is the protective fluid for all tissues of the oral cavity. It protects the soft tissues from abrasion by rough materials and from chemicals. It allows for the continuous mineralisation of the tooth enamel after eruption and helps in remineralisation of the enamel in the early stages of dental caries. Saliva is an aqueous fluid with 1% organic and inorganic materials. The major determinant of the salivary composition is the flow rate which in turn depends upon three factors: the time of day, the type of stimulus, and the degree of stimulation. The salivary pH ranges from 5.5 to 7 depending on the flow rate. At high flow rates, the sodium and bicarbonate concentrations increase leading to an increase in the pH. The daily salivary volume is between 0.5 to 2 liters and it is this amount of fluid that is available to hydrate oral mucosal dosage forms. A main reason behind the selection of hydrophilic polymeric matrices as vehicles for oral transmucosal drug delivery systems is this water rich environment of the oral cavity.

3.3 ORAL MUCOSAL PERMEATION ENHANCERS

Similar to any other mucosal membrane, the buccal mucosa as a site for drug delivery has limitations as well. One of the major disadvantages associated with buccal drug delivery is the low flux which results in low drug bioavailability. Various compounds have been investigated for their use as buccal penetration enhancers in order to increase the flux of drugs through the mucosa as shown in Table (1).

Table 1. List of compounds used as oral mucosal permeation enhancers.

Permeation Enhancer	
23-lauryl ether.	Methyloleate.
Aprotinin.	Oleic acid.
Azone.	Phosphatidylcholine.
Benzalkonium chloride.	Polyoxyethylene.
Cetylpyridinium chloride.	Polysorbate 80.
Cetyltrimethylammonium	Sodium EDTA.
Bromide.	Sodium glycocholate.
Cyclodextrin.	Sodium glycodeoxycholate.
Dextran sulfate.	Sodium lauryl sulfate.
Lauric acid.	Sodium salicylate.
Lauric acid/Propylene glycol	Sodium taurocholate.
Lysophosphatidylcholine.	Sodium taurodeoxycholate
Menthol.	Sulfoxides.
Methoxysalicylate.	Various alkyl glycosides.

MECHANISMS OF ACTION OF PERMEATION ENHANCERS.

Mechanisms by which penetration enhancers are thought to improve mucosal absorption are as follows. Also summrised in Table (2)

1) Changing mucus rheology

Mucus forms viscoelastic layer of varying thickness that affects drug absorption. Further, saliva covering the mucus layers also hinders the absorption. Some permeation enhancers' act by reducing the viscosity of the mucus and saliva overcomes this barrier.

2) Increasing the fluidity of lipid bilayer membrane

The most accepted mechanism of drug absorption through buccal mucosa is intracellular route. Some enhancers disturb the intracellular lipid packing by interaction with either lipid packing by interaction with either lipid or protein components.

3) Acting on the components at tight junctions

Some enhancers act on desmosomes, a major component at the tight junctions there by increases drug absorption.

4) By overcoming the enzymatic barrier

These act by inhibiting the various peptidases and proteases present within buccal mucosa, thereby overcoming the enzymatic barrier. In addition, changes in membrane fluidity also alter the enzymatic activity indirectly.

5) Increasing the thermodynamic activity of drugs

Some enhancers increase the solubility of drug there by alters the partition coefficient. This leads to increased thermodynamic activity resulting better absorption.

3.4 THEORIES OF MUCOADHESION

The phenomena of bioadhesion occurs by a complex mechanism. Till date, six theories have been proposed which can improve our understanding for the phenomena of adhesion and can also be extended to explain the mechanism of bioadhesion. The theories include: (a) the electronic theory, (b) the wetting theory, (c) the adsorption theory, (d) the diffusion theory, (e) the mechanical theory and (f) the cohesive theory. The electronic theory proposes transfer of electrons amongst the surfaces resulting in the formation of an electrical double layer thereby giving rise to attractive forces. The wetting theory postulates that if the contact angle of liquids on the substrate surface is lower, then there is a greater affinity for the liquid to the substrate surface. If two such substrate surfaces are brought in contact with each other in the presence of the liquid, the liquid may act as an adhesive amongst the substrate surfaces. The adsorption theory proposes the presence of intermolecular forces, viz. hydrogen bonding and Van der Waal's forces, for the adhesive interaction amongst the substrate surfaces. The diffusion theory assumes the diffusion of the polymer chains, present on the substrate surfaces, across the adhesive interface thereby forming a networked structure. The mechanical theory explains the diffusion of the liquid adhesives into the micro-cracks and irregularities present on the substrate surface thereby forming an interlocked structure which gives rise to adhesion. The cohesive theory proposes that the phenomena of bioadhesion are mainly due to the intermolecular interactions amongst like-molecules.

Table 2: Mucosal penetration enhancers and mechanisms of action.

Slno	Classification	Examples	Mechanism
1	Surfactants	Anionic: sodium lauryl, sodium lauryl Cationic: cetylpyridinium chloride Nonionic: poloxamer, Brij, Span, Myrj, Tween Bile Salts: Sodium glycolate, sodium taurodeoxycholate, sodium taurocholate Azone	Perturbation of intercellular lipids, protein domain integrity
2	Fatty acids	oleic acid, caprylic acid	Increase fluidity of phospholipid domains
3	Cyclodextrins	α, β, γ cyclodextrin, methyllated β-cyclodextrins	Inclusion of membrane compounds
4	Chelators	EDTA, Sodium citrate	interfere with ca polycrylates
5	Positively charged polymers	:Chitosan, trimethyl chitosan	Ionic interaction with negative charge on the mucosal surface
6	Cationic compounds	Ply-L-arginine, L-lysine	Ionic interaction with negative charge on the mucosal surface

Based on the above theories, the process of bioadhesion can be broadly classified into two categories, namely chemical (electronic and adsorption theories) and physical (wetting, diffusion and cohesive theory) methods. The process of adhesion may be divided into two stages. During the first stage (also known as contact stage), wetting of mucoadhesive polymer and mucous membrane occurs followed by the consolidation stage, where the physico-chemical interactions prevail.

As mentioned above, bioadhesion may take place either by physical or by chemical interactions. These interactions can be further classified as hydrogen bonds, Van der Waals force and hydrophobic bonds which are considered as physical interactions while the formation of ionic and covalent bonds are categorized as chemical interactions. Hydrogen bonds are formed due to the interaction of the electronegative and electropositive atoms though there is no actual transfer of electrons. Example of this kind of interaction includes formation of gelled structure when aqueous solutions of polyvinyl alcohol and glycine are mixed. Van der Waals forces are either due to presence of the dipole-dipole interactions in polar molecules or due to the dispersion forces amongst non-polar substrates. Hydrophobic bonds are formed due to the interaction of the non-polar groups when the polymers are dispersed in an aqueous solution. Freeze-thawing of polyvinyl alcohol solution in water exhibits this kind of interaction. Ionic bonds are formed due to the electrostatic interactions amongst the polymers (e.g. instantaneous formation of gelled structure when alginate and chitosan solutions in water are mixed) while covalent bonds are formed due to the sharing of electrons amongst the atoms (e.g. crosslinking reaction amongst genipin and amino groups).

The phenomena of bioadhesion occurs by a complex mechanism. Till date, six theories have been proposed which can improve our understanding for the phenomena of adhesion and can also be extended to explain the mechanism of bioadhesion. The theories include: (a) the electronic theory, (b) the wetting theory, (c) the adsorption theory, (d) the diffusion theory, (e) the mechanical theory and (f) the cohesive theory. The electronic theory proposes transfer of electrons amongst the surfaces resulting in the formation of an electrical double layer thereby giving rise to attractive forces. The wetting theory postulates that if the contact angle of liquids on the substrate surface is lower, then there is a greater affinity for the liquid to the substrate surface. If two such substrate surfaces are brought in contact with each other in the presence of the liquid, the liquid may act as an adhesive amongst the substrate surfaces. The adsorption theory proposes the presence of intermolecular forces, viz. hydrogen bonding and Van der Waal's forces, for the adhesive interaction amongst the substrate surfaces. The diffusion theory assumes the diffusion of the polymer chains, present on the substrate surfaces, across the adhesive interface thereby forming a networked structure. The mechanical theory explains the diffusion of the liquid adhesives into the micro-cracks and irregularities present on the substrate surface thereby forming an interlocked structure which gives rise to adhesion. The cohesive theory proposes that the phenomena of bioadhesion are mainly due to the intermolecular interactions amongst like-molecules.

Based on the above theories, the process of bioadhesion can be broadly classified into two categories, namely chemical (electronic and adsorption theories) and physical (wetting, diffusion and cohesive theory) methods. The process of adhesion may be divided into two stages. During the first stage (also known as contact stage), wetting of mucoadhesive polymer and mucous membrane occurs followed by the consolidation stage, where the physico-chemical interactions prevail.

As mentioned above, bioadhesion may take place either by physical or by chemical interactions. These interactions can be further classified as hydrogen bonds, Van der Waals force and hydrophobic bonds which are considered as physical interactions while the formation of ionic and covalent bonds are categorized as chemical interactions. Hydrogen bonds are formed due to the interaction of the electronegative and electropositive atoms though there is no actual transfer of electrons. Example of this kind of interaction includes formation of gelled structure when aqueous solutions of polyvinyl alcohol and glycine are mixed. Van der Waals forces are either due to presence of the dipole-dipole interactions in polar molecules or due to the dispersion forces amongst non-polar substrates. Hydrophobic bonds are formed due to the interaction of the non-polar groups when the polymers are dispersed in an aqueous solution. Freeze-thawing of polyvinyl alcohol solution in water exhibits this kind of interaction. Ionic bonds are formed due to the electrostatic interactions amongst the polymers (e.g. instantaneous formation of gelled structure when alginate and chitosan solutions in water are mixed) while covalent bonds are formed due to the sharing of electrons amongst the atoms (e.g. crosslinking reaction amongst genipin and amino groups).

SITES FOR MUCOADHESIVE DRUG DELIVERY SYSTEMS

The common sites of application where mucoadhesive polymers have the ability to delivery pharmacologically active agents include oral cavity, eye conjunctiva, vagina, nasal cavity and gastrointestinal tract. The current section of the review will give an overview of the above-mentioned delivery sites.

The buccal cavity has a very limited surface area of around 50 cm^2 but the easy access to the site makes it a preferred location for delivering active agents. The site provides an opportunity to deliver pharmacologically active agents systemically by avoiding hepatic first-pass metabolism in addition to the local treatment of the oral lesions. The sublingual mucosa is relatively more permeable than the buccal mucosa (due to the presence of large number of smooth muscle and immobile mucosa), hence formulations for sublingual delivery are designed to release the active agent quickly while mucoadhesive formulation is of importance for the delivery of active agents to the buccal mucosa where the active agent has to be released in a controlled manner. This makes the buccal cavity more suitable for mucoadhesive drug delivery. The various mucoadhesive polymers used for the development of buccal delivery systems include cyanoacrylates, polyacrylic acid, sodium carboxymethylcellulose, hyaluronic acid, hydroxypropylcellulose, polycarbophil, chitosan and gellan. The delivery systems are generally coated with a drug and water impermeable film so as to prevent the washing of the active agent by the saliva.

Like buccal cavity, nasal cavity also provides a potential site for the development of formulations where mucoadhesive polymers can play an important role. The nasal mucosal layer has a surface area of around 150-200 cm^2. The residence time of a particulate matter in the nasal mucosa varies between 15 and 30 min, which have been attributed to the increased activity of the mucociliary layer in the presence of foreign particulate matter. The polymers used in the development of formulations for the development of nasal delivery system include copolymer of methyl vinyl ether, hydroxypropylmethylcellulose, sodium carboxymethylcellulose, carbopol-934P and Eudragit RL-100.

Due to the continuous formation of tears and blinking of eye lids there is a rapid removal of the active medicament from the ocular cavity, which results in the poor bioavailability of the active agents. This can be minimized by delivering the drugs using ocular insert or patches. The mucoadhesive polymers used for the ocular delivery include thiolated poly(acrylic acid), poloxamer, celluloseacetophthalate, methyl cellulose, hydroxy ethyl cellulose, poly(amidoamine) dendrimers, poly(dimethyl siloxane) and poly (vinyl pyrrolidone).

The vaginal and the rectal lumen have also been explored for the delivery of the active agents both systemically and locally. The active agents meant for the systemic delivery by this route of administration bypasses the hepatic first-pass metabolism. Quite often the delivery systems suffer from migration within the vaginal/rectal lumen which might affect the delivery of the active agent to the specific location. The use of mucoadhesive polymers for the development of delivery system helps in reducing the migration of the same thereby promoting better therapeutic efficacy. The polymers used in the development of vaginal and rectal delivery systems include mucin, gelatin, polycarbophil and poloxamer.

Gastrointestinal tract is also a potential site which has been explored since long for the development of mucoadhesive based formulations. The modulation of the transit time of the delivery systems in a particular location of the gastrointestinal system by using mucoadhesive polymers has generated much interest among researchers around the world. The various mucoadhesive polymers which have been used for the development of oral delivery systems include chitosan, poly (acrylic acid), alginate, poly (methacrylic acid) and sodium carboxymethyl cellulose.

POLYMERS IN MUCOSAL DRUG DELIVERY

Mucoadhesive delivery systems are being explored for the localization of the active agents to a particular location/ site. Polymers have played an important role in designing such systems so as to increase the residence time of the active agent at the desired location. Polymers used in mucosal delivery system may be of natural or synthetic origin. In this section we will briefly discuss some of the common classes of mucoadhesive polymers.

Hydrophilic polymers

Hydrophilic polymers are those containing carboxylic group e.:hibit the best mucoadhesive properties, polyvinyl pyrrolidone (PVP), Methylcellulose (MC), Sodium carboxy methylcellulose(SCMC) Hydroxy propyl cellulose (HPC) and other cellulose derivative.

The polymers within this category are soluble in water. Matrices developed with these polymers swell when put into an aqueous media with subsequent dissolution of the matrix. The polyelectrolytes extend greater mucoadhesive property when compared with neutral polymers Anionic polyelectrolytes, e.g. poly (acrylic acid) and carboxymethyl cellulose, have been extensively used for designing mucoadhesive delivery systems due to their ability to exhibit strong hydrogen bonding with the mucin present in the mucosal layer. Chitosan provides an excellent example of cationic polyelectrolyte, which has been extensively used for developing mucoadhesive polymer due to its good biocompatibility and biodegradable properties. Chitosan undergoes electrostatic interactions with the negatively charged mucin chains thereby exhibiting mucoadhesive property. The ionic polymers may be used to develop ionic complex with the counter-ionic drug molecules so as to have a drug delivery matrix exhibiting mucoadhesive property. In a recent study, partially neutralized poly (acrylic acid) complex was developed in the presence of levobetaxolol hydrochloride, a potent cardiac β-blocker. The delivery system was prone to dissolution as the time progressed due to the release of the incorporated drug. Mucoadhesive microcapsules can be designed with same principle by using orifice-ionic gelation method. This technique has been used to design a delivery system of gliclazide, an anti-diabetic drug, using sodium alginate, sodium carboxymethyl cellulose, carbopol 934P and hydroxy propylmethyl cellulose. The delivery system showed the release of gliclazide for an extended period of time due to its mucoadhesive properties. Non-ionic polymers, e.g. poloxamer, hydroxypropyl methyl cellulose, methyl cellulose, poly (vinyl alcohol) and poly (vinyl pyrrolidone), have also been used for mucoadhesive properties. The hydrophilic polymers form viscous solutions when dissolved in water and hence may also be used as viscosity modifying/enhancing agents in the development of liquid ocular delivery systems so as to increase the bioavailability of the active agents by reducing the drainage of the administered formulations. These polymers may be directly compressed in the presence of drugs so as to have a mucoadhesive delivery system.

Numerous polysaccharides and its derivatives like chitosan, methyl cellulose, hyaluronic acid, hydroxypropyl methylcellulose, hydroxypropyl cellulose, xanthan gum, gellan gum, guar gum, and carrageenan have found applications in ocular mucoadhesive delivery systems. Cellulose and its derivates have been reported to have surface active property in addition to its film forming capability. Cellulose derivatives with lower surface acting property are generally preferred in ocular delivery systems as they cause reduced eye irritation. Of the various cellulose derivates, sodium carboxymethyl cellulose has been found to have excellent ocular mucoadhesive property. Cationic cellulose derivatives (e.g. cationic hydroxyethyl celluloses) have been used in conjunction with various anionic polymers for the development of sustained delivery systems.

Hydrogels

Hyrogels are the class of polymeric biomaterial that exhibit the basic characteristics of an hydrogels to swell by absorbing water interacting by means of adhesion with the mucus that covers epithelia i.e.

- Anionic group - Carbopol, Polyacrylates and their crosslinked modifications
- Cationic group - Chitosan and its derivatives
- Neutral group -   Eudragit- NE30D etc.

Hydrogels can be defined as three-dimensionally crosslinked polymer chains which have the ability to hold water within its porous structure. The water holding capacity of the hydrogels is mainly due to the presence of hydrophilic functional groups like hydroxyl, amino and carboxyl groups. In general, with the increase in the crosslinking density there is an associated decrease in the mucoadhesion. Thielmann et al. reported the thermal crosslinking of poly (acrylic acid) and methyl cellulose. They reported that with the increase in the crosslinking density, there was a reduction in the solubility parameters and swelling which resulted in a reduction of mucoadhesion. Hydrogels prepared by the condensation reaction of poly (acrylic acid) and sucrose indicated an increase in the mucoadhesive property with the increase in the crosslinking density and was attributed to increase in the poly (acrylic acid) chain density per unit area. Acrylates have been used to develop mucoadhesive delivery systems which have the ability to deliver peptide bioactive agents to the upper small intestine region without any change in the bioactivity of the peptides. In a typical experimentation, Wood and Peppas developed a system in which ethylene glycol chains were grafted on methacrylic acid hydrogels and were subsequently functionalized with wheat germ agglutinin. Wheat germ agglutinin helped in improving the intestinal residence time of the delivery system by binding with the specific carbohydrate moieties present in the intestinal mucosa. In addition to the drug targeting, mucoadhesive hydrogel based formulations for improving the bioavailability of the poorly water soluble drug. Muller and Jacobs prepared a nanosuspension of buparvaquone, a poorly water soluble drug, by incorporating it within carbopol and chitosan based hydrogels. The mucoadhesive delivery systems showed improved bioavailability of the drug when compared over the nanosuspension. This was attributed to the increased retention time of the delivery system within the gastrointestinal tract.

Thiolated polymers

The presence of free thiol groups in the polymeric skeleton helps in the formation of disulphide bonds with that of the cysteine-rich sub-domains present in mucin which can substantially improve the mucoadhesive properties of the polymers (e.g. poly (acrylic acid) and chitosan) in addition to the paracellular uptake of the bioactive agents. Various thiolated polymers include chitosan–iminothiolane, poly(acrylic acid)–cysteine, poly(acrylic acid)–homocysteine, chitosan–thioglycolic acid, chitosan–thioethylamidine, alginate–cysteine, poly(methacrylic acid)–cysteine and sodium carboxymethylcellulose–cysteine.

Lectin-based polymers

Lectins are proteins which have the ability to reversibly bind with specific sugar / carbohydrate residues and are found in both animal and plant kingdom in addition to various microorganisms. Many lectins have been found to be toxic and immunogenic which may lead to systemic anaphylaxis in susceptible individuals on subsequent exposure. The specific affinity of lectins towards sugar or carbohydrate residues provides them with specific cyto-adhesive property and is being explored to develop targeted delivery systems. Lectins extracted from legumes have been widely explored for targeted delivery systems. The various lectins which have shown specific binding to the mucosa include lectins extracted from Ulex europaeus I, soybean, peanut and Lens culinarius. The use of wheat germ agglutinin has been on the rise due to its least immunogenic reactions, amongst available lectins, in addition to its capability to bind to the intestinal and alveolar epithelium and hence could be used to design oral and aerosol delivery systems.

3.5 MECHANISIM OF BIOADHESION

The phenomenon of bioadhesion of the polymer depends upon its physicochemical properties. Some of the physicochemical factors of mucoadhesive polymers are as follows:

➢ Hydrohillic molecules containing several hydrogen bond forming groups.

➢ Surface tension characteristics suitable for wetting mucous / mucosal tissues surface.

➢ The polymers containing carboxyl group which are anionic in nature.

➢ Polymers which have molecular weight greater than 100,000.

➢ Sufficient flexibility to penetrate the mucosal network or tissues crevices.

The different mechanism of polymer / substrate interaction the bond formation the mucoadhesives are the electronic, adsorption, wetting, diffusion, and fracture theories.

1) Wetting theory

This theory is applicable to liquid bioadhesive system. It is based on the ability of a liquid or paste to spread over a biological system. The ability of adhesive to spread on mucin influence the intimate contact between mucoadhesive and mucin. The thermodynamic work of adhesion is a function of surface tension of surface in contact as well as interfacial tension.

2) Diffusion theory

The diffusion theory describes the interpretation of the mucoadhesive (polymer) and the substrate (mucin) to a sufficient depth and creation of a semipermenant adhesive bond. In bioadhesion, the polymer first brought into contact with the mucous, and over time, the concentration gradient across the interface causes the diffusion of chains of the bioadhesive into the mucous layer and also the diffusion of glycoprotein chains of mucous into the bioadhesive polymer. The rate of the diffusion is dependant on the chemical potential gradient and the diffusion coeffient of macro molecules through a cross linked network.

Despite the interdiffusion in compatible polymers as been demonstrated by radiometric studies,the exact depth of penetration required to achieve adequate mucoadhesion is not known, However the mean diffusional path length(S),can be derived as

$$S = (2tD)^{1/2}$$

Where D is the diffusion coefficient.

3) Electronic theory

The mucin glycoprotein and mucoadhesive polymer posses different electronic structures, therefore the electronic tranafer is likely to occur when contact is made. This electronic transfer results in formation of electrical double layer at the adhesive interface with subsequent adhesion. Hence, the adhesive / mucin interface can be treated as capacitor, which tends to be charged when the two surfaces are in close contactand discharged when they are separated.

4) Adsorption Theory

The attachment of adhesive to biological tissues on the basis of a group of interactions know as "secondary forces" The vander waals forces attraction are the sum of all attractions between uncharged molecules. These attractive forces arrives from,

Polar or keesom forces developed due to orientation of permanent dipoles in two molecules.

Induction debye forces developed due to induce dipole and permanent dipole.

Dispersion or London forces developed due to changes in the charge distribution around non polar molecule

Hydrogen bonding developed between two the nonpolar, due to the tendancy of water molecules to exclude non polar molecules or between the ionized carboxyl groups or surfaces.

5) Fracture Theory

This Theory describe force require to separate two surface after adhesion

Maximum tensile strength (Sm) produce during detachment can be determine by dividing max. force of detachment (Fm) by total surface area(Ao)

$$Sm = Fm/Ao$$

In uniform single – component system , Fracture strength (sf) which is equal to the max. stress of detachment (sm) is proportional to fracture energy (gc)

$$Sf = (yc\ E/C)1/2$$

E = Young's modules of elasticity.

C = critical crack strength   yc = fracture energy .

Formulations of buccal bioadhesive drug delivery:

The development and the use of fast dissolving dosage form in therapeutic practice have shown that buccal administration is clinically feasible. However, the clinical success of oral mucosal drug delivery depends on the ability of the drug delivery system to achieve, and to maintain the therapeutic levels for a define period of time. An the oral mucosal drug delivery system must be able to deliver an adequate amount of drug according to desire absorption profile (rate and duration). The availability of this amount of drug mainly depends on the formulation factors of the drug delivery system. Therefore, the drug release pattern from the delivery system is crucial and must be carefully consider. Fig-2 shows the different design of buccal delivery systems various dosage form for oral mucosal drug delivery. Some commercial buccal bioadhesive drug delivery system are listed in table.

Table 3: Dosage forms developed for the buccal mucosal drug delivery and some commercially available bioadhesive formulations

Dosage for developed	Commercially available bioadhesive buccal delivery system.
Solution, tablets, lyophilized tablet, chewing gum, bioadhesive tablets, solution-spray, laminated systems and patches, hydrogels, adhesive film, hollow fibre, microsperes, liposomes	Bioadhesive tablet :- Sublingual mucosal delivery of nitro glycerine : Susadrin® Buccal mucosal delivery of prochlroperazine : Buccastem® Chewing gum :- Buccal mucosal delivery of nicotine: Nicorette®

Dosage for developed Commercially available bioadhesive buccal delivery system.

Solution, tablets, lyophilized tablet, chewing gum, bioadhesive tablets, solution-spray, laminated systems and patches, hydrogels, adhesive film, hollow fibre, microsperes, liposomes Bioadhesive tablet :- Sublingual mucosal delivery of nitro glycerine : Susadrin® Buccal mucosal delivery of prochlroperazine : Buccastem® Chewing gum :- Buccal mucosal delivery of nicotine Nicorette®

Bioadhesive tablets

Bioadhesive tablets are immobilized drug delivery system. They can be formulated into monolithic, partially coated or multi-layered matrices. Monolithic tablets are esay to manufacture by conventional techniques and provide for the possibility of loading large amount of drug. Drug can be coincorporated with an absorption enhancer, if required. Partial coatingof monolithic tablet affords protection of every face of tablet, which is not in contact mucosa. Such systems allow undirected drug release and avoid drug release into salivary fluids. Fig-3 is showing the possible designs of buccal bioadhesive drug delivery. Multi-layered tablets cotd be of a variety of geometrical arrangements. In case of bi-layered tablets, drug can be incorporated in the adhesive layer, which comes in contact with the mucosal surface. This drug containing mucoadhesive layer is then protected from the oral cavity environment by a second upper inert layer, which faces into the oral cavity. Alternatively, the drug can be incorporated into the upper non-adhesive layer to release the drug into oral cavity.

Retention of an oral mucosal drug delivery system is a requirement for the use of the oral mucosa as platform, for prolonged drug delivery. The use of cellubsic or acrylic polymers generally offers almost immediate, high adhesion performance for prolonged period of time, even with high drug content. Factors such as nature of polymer, the drug/polymer ratio and swelling kinetics influence the drug release from bioadhesive tablets. The imitations of buccal tablets are;

- The small surface of contact with mucosa

- Their lack of feasibility

- It is difficult to obtain high release rates, which is required for some drugs

- The extent and frequency of contact may cause irritation following chronic application on the buccal and sublingual mucosa.

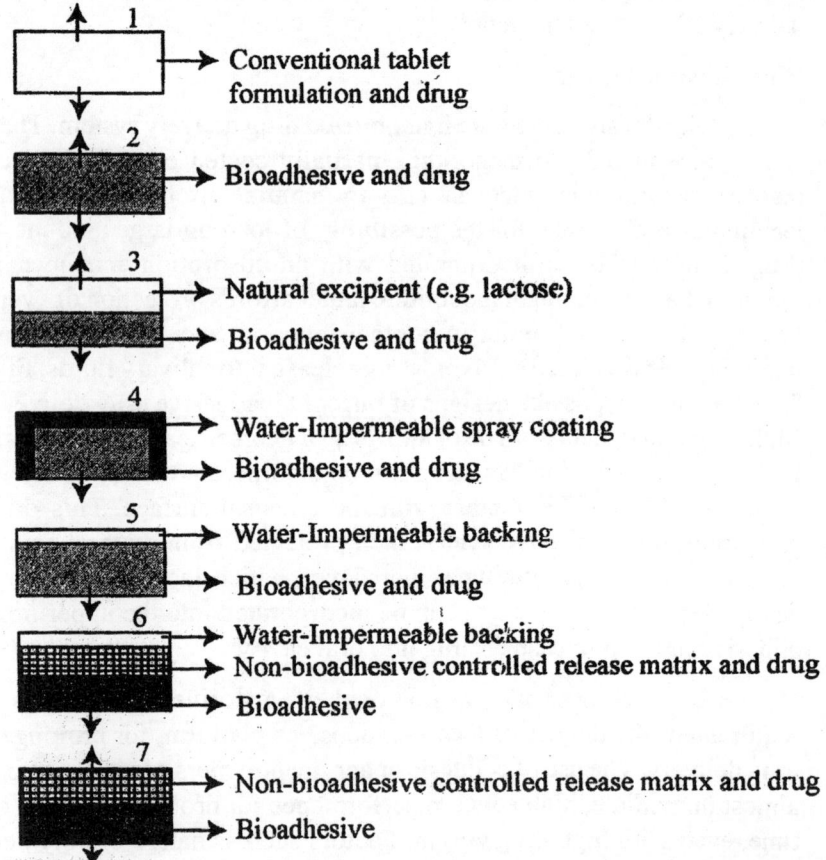

Fig.2: **Possible design of Buccal delivery systems including bioadhesive for systemic Drug Delivery.**

The adhesive tablets were developed into a system releasing triamcinolone acetonide ointment to treat aphthous stomatitis. The system is commercially available, named Aftach®, a small, thin, double layered tablet. The upper layer consists of and serves as a supportive layer and lower adhesive layer consists of drug, hydroxyl propylcellulose and carbopol 934. Bottenberg et al., examined the use of various polymers in the preparation of noral slow-release tablets containing fluoride for the treatment of dental caries. Modified starch, poly (acrylic acid) (PPA), poly (ethylene glycol) (PEG) and sodium carboxy methylcellulose were the bioadhesive polymers investigated. A modified maize starch tablet containing 5% PPA and PEG with a 300,000 dalton molecular weight proved to be the most successful formulation. Buccoadhesive matrix tablets containing hydrocortisone hemisuccinate were developed by using various polymers (hydroxyl propyl cellulose, hydroxyl propyl methyl cellulose, polycarbophil and modified maize starch). The maize starch formulation demonstrated the optimal gingival tolerance, delivered hydrocortisone *in vitro* up to 24hrs, dissolved and eventually resulted in the complete erosion of tablet.

3.6 EVALUATION OF BIOADHESIVE DRUG DELIVERY SYSTEMS

In *vitro* Evaluation of various bioadhesive polymers.

> **Shear Stress Measurement of Bioadhesive Polymers**

Two smooth, polished plexi glass blocked are selected one box was fixed the adhesive ' Araldite' on a glass plate, which is fixed on the leveled table. The level is adjusted with the a spirit lamp. To the upper blocked the thread is tied and the thread is passed down through a pulley. The length of the thread from the pulley to pan is 12cms.at the end of the thread a pan weight 17g is attached into which the weights can be added. Different polymer solution of 3% w/v strength are prepared using water as solvent. A fixed amount (one drop) of polymer solution is kept on the center of the first block with a pipette and then the second block is placed on the first block and pressed by applying 100g weight such that the drop of polymer spreads as uniform film in between the two blocks. After keeping it for fixed time intervals of 5, 10, 15 and 30 min, the weights are added to pan. The weights are just sufficient to pull the upper block or to make it slide down from the base block represent the adhesion strength, ie the shear stress required.

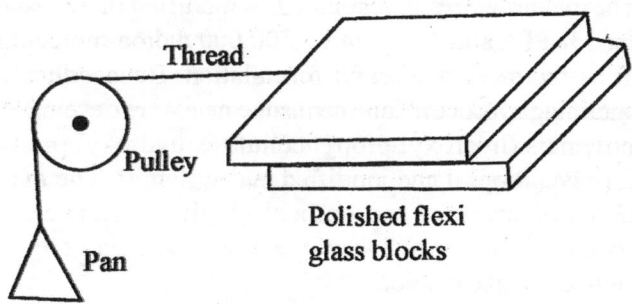

Fig.3: Shear stress measurement of boiadhesive polymers.

> **Detachment Force Measurement:**

This method is to measure in vitro mucoadhesive capacity of different polymers. It is a modified method developed by Martti Marvola to assess the tendency of mucoadhesive to adhere to esophagus. It consist of a single organ bath, a stand, glass rod, apan for keeping beaker and a reservoir for addition of water into beaker. In these method, immediately after slaughter, the intestine is remove from, the sleep and transported to laboratory in tyrode solution(composition :sodium chloride – 8g/L, potassium chloride – 0.2g\L, calcium ehloride. 2H2O- 0.134g/L, sodium bicarbonate 1g/L, sodium di hydrogen phosphate 0.05g/L and glucose H2O 1g/L). During the experiment the solution is aerated with pure oxygen and kept at 37°c. Segments of 6-7 cm long are cut from the intestine. The lower end of the intestine segment is tied off then tied to the aerator tube and the upper is tied around the glass tube of diameter of 15mm as shown in the fig.

For example, 6mm plane tablet, tablet layered on one side with mucoadhesive polymer and polymer matrix (2:1ratio) tablet of the given drug were prepared. A fine hole drilled in the tablet to be tested with the fine needle at the centre. A thread was passed through it and tied around the tablet. The other end of the thread to the glass rod suspended from the stand. The length of the thread was such that in resting stage the tablet should be in at the middle of the intestinal piece. To the other end of the glass rod a pan was tied in which a beaker was placed. After inserting the tablet into intestinal segment and lightly presssing intestinal segment with tablet by a forceps. The assemble should be kept undisturbed for a fix time interval of 30min and 1 hr. than water was added with a burette slowly drop by drop into the beaker. The amount of water requied to pull out the tablet from the intestinal segment represents the force required to pull the tablet against the adhesion. The force in Newton is calculated by the equation,

$$F = 0.00981 \ W/2$$

Where, W is the amount of water.

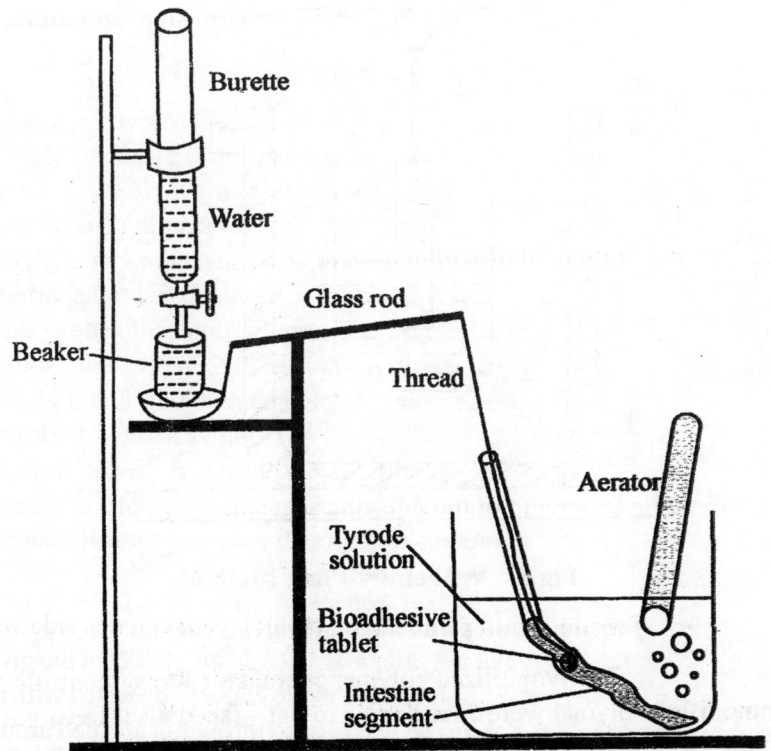

Fig.4: Assembly developed for detachment force measurement

> **Wilhelmly Plate Technique**

This technique was traditional been used for dynamic contact angle measurement and involves a microbalance or tensiometer. A glass slide is coated with polymer of interest and than dip into the beaker of synthetic or natural mucous. The surface tension, contact angle and adhesive force can be automatically measured using available software.

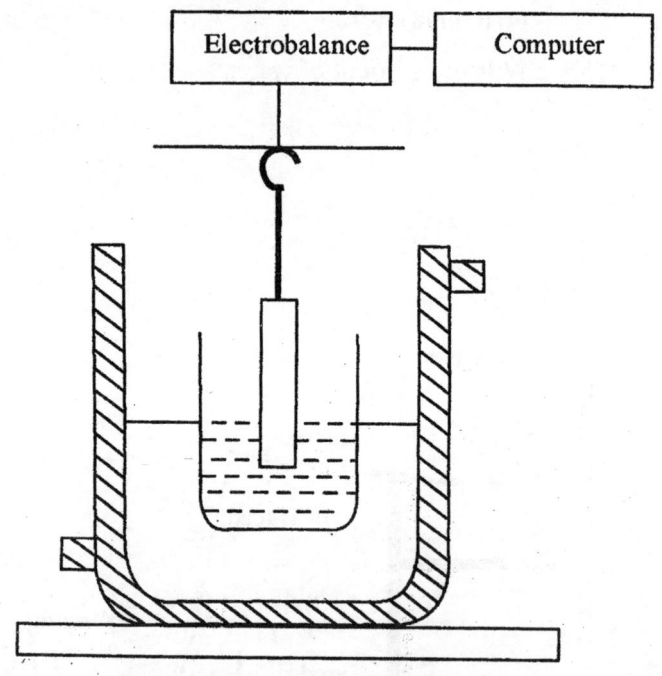

Fig.5: Wilhelmly Plate Method

> **Tensile Studies on Mucoadhesive Polymer Conjugates:**

The lyophilized polymer conjugate (30mg), controls and unmodified polymer were compressed to flat – faced disc. Tensiometer studies with this disc were carried on native porcine intestinal mucosa. Test discs were therefore, attached to the mucosa with a force of 2.5mN. after contact time between test disc and mucosa of 30min in 100mM

Tris-HCl buffered saline (TBS) pH 6.8 at 25°C, the mucosa was pulled at a rate of 0.1mm s^{-1} from the disc. The total work of adhesion (TWA) representing the area under the force/ distance curve and the maximum detachment force(MDF) were determined using the WINWEDGE software in combination with EXCEL 5.0(a Microsoft software).

> **Mucoadhesive Studies**

In order to evaluate the binding to the mucosa as well as the cohesiveness of the tablet, and appropriate new method has been established. The prepared tablets (flat-surface discs) were attached to freshly excised intestinal porcine in mucosa, which has been spanned on a stainless steel cylinder (diameter:4.4cm, height:5.5cm, apparatus:4-cylinders,USP XXII).

Thereafter, the cylinder was placed in the dissolution apparatus according the USP containing 100mM TBS pH 6.8 at 37±0.5°C. The fully immersed cylinder was agitated with 250 rpm. The detachment, disintegration and /or erosion of test tablets were observed and recorded within time period of 10hr.

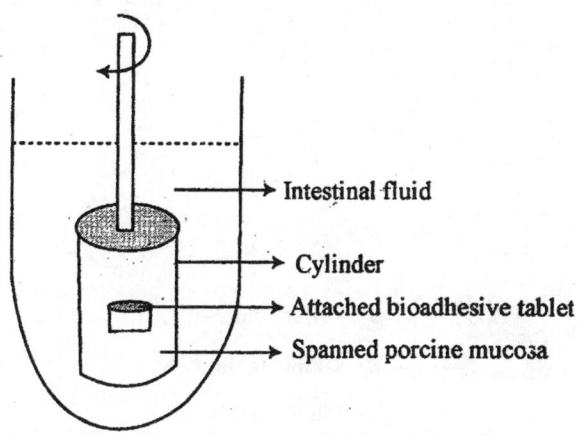

Fig.6: The test system for evaluation of mucoadhesion of bioadhesive tablet.

➢ **Adhesion Force Measurement**

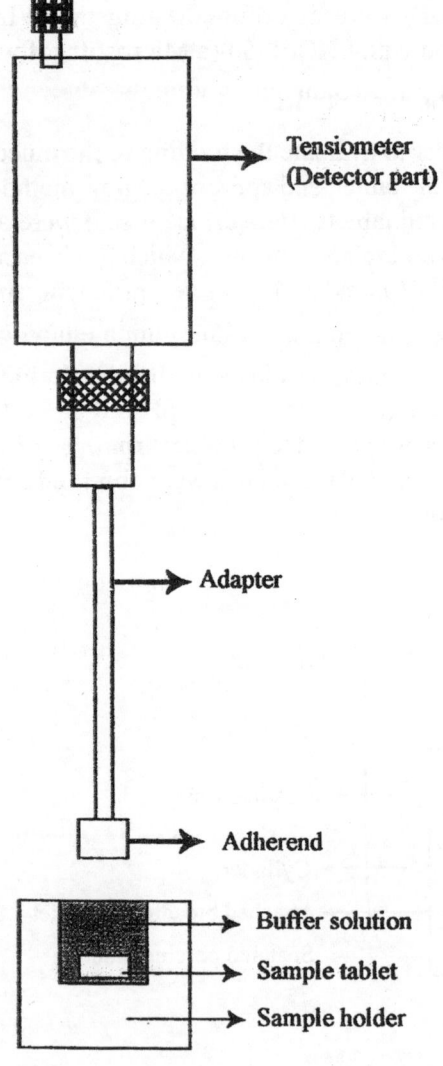

Fig.7: Schematic representation of experimental setup for determination of bioadhesion force.

The adhesion properties of bioadhesive polymer tablets can be evaluated by measuring the force required to separate the tablet from an adherend. The tablet is attached to the holder to the cyanoacrylate type adhesives. Buffer solutions (2ml;pH 2.0,3.5 and 5.0)are gently added on the tablet to hydrate the tablet surface for 5 min at 25^0C. Othewise a lyophilized porcine dermis and rabbit peritoneal membrane excised from male New Zealand white rabbits(3.0-3.5kg) are used as adherends. The rabbits are killed by pentobarbital injection, the peritoneal membrane is extracted and stored at -10^0c.before the experiment, it is thawed at 4^0c in an isotonic saline solution. The residual water on the surface is removed with the help of filter paper. The porcine dermis of rabbit peritoneal membrane, which is cut into round shape with a diameter of 5mm,is attached to the tip of adapter in tensiometer with a cyanoacrylate type adhesive. The adherends are the immersed in the buffer solutions (pH 2.0,3.5, and 5.0) for 5 minutes at 25^0 c before the measurement. The holder wearing the sample tablet is then lifted up in contact with adherent, which is preliminarily hydrated in buffer solutions by applying a loading pressure of 250 gm/cm^2 .the tablet and the adherend are kept in contact with each other for 3 min. The tablet is then streched from the adherend at an extension rate of 4mm/s and the force required to detach the tablet from the adherend is recorded.

3.7 IN VIVO METHODS

In vivo methods were first originated by Beckett and Triggs with the so-called buccal absorption test. Using this method, the kinetics of drug absorption were measured. The methodology involves the swirling of a 25 ml sample of the test solution for up to 15 minutes by human volunteers followed by the expulsion of the solution. The amount of drug remaining in the expelled volume is then determined in order to assess the amount of drug absorbed. The drawbacks of this method include salivary dilution of the drug, accidental swallowing of a portion of the sample solution, and the inability to localize the drug solution within a specific site (buccal, sublingual, or gingival) of the oral cavity. Various modifications of the buccal absorption test have been carried out correcting for salivary dilution and accidental swallowing, but these modifications also suffer from the inability of site localization. A feasible approach to achieve absorption site localization is to retain the drug on the buccal mucosa using a bioadhesive system. Pharmacokinetic parameters such as bioavailability can then be calculated from the plasma concentration vs. time profile

Other in vivo methods include those carried out using a small perfusion chamber attached to the upper lip of anesthetized dogs. The perfusion chamber is attached to the tissue by cyanoacrylate cement. The drug solution is circulated through the device for a predetermined period of time and sample fractions are then collected from the perfusion chamber (to determine the amount of drug remaining in the chamber) and blood samples are drawn after 0 and 30 minutes (to determine amount of drug absorbed across the mucosa).

REVIEW QUESTIONS

ESSAY QUESTIONS

1. a. Write Advantages and Disadvantages of Mucoadhesive Drug Delivery Systems?
    b. what is the mechanism of bioadhesion and its invitro evaluation?
2. a. What criteria should be followed in polymer selection for Mucoadhesive Drug Delivery Systems?
    b. Write a note on invitro wash off test?
3. What are in vitro and In-vivo Evaluation techniques for Mucoadhesive Drug Delivery Systems?
4. What are various approaches for the formulation of Mucoadhesive Drug Delivery Systems?

SHORT QUESTIONS

1. Write a note on polymer use in mucoadhesive drug delivery system.
2. Give a detailed explanation on theories involved in mucoadhesion and bioadhesion.
3. Which are the permeation enhancers used in mucoadhesive drug delivery system and give its mechanism.

Chapter 4

TARGETED DRUG DELIVERY SYSTEMS

4.1 LIPOSOMES

Liposomes have been widely investigated since 1970 as drug carriers for improving the delivery of therapeutic agents to specific sites in the body. Liposomes are most developed nana carriers for novel and targeted drug delivery. As a result, numerous improvements have been made, thus making this technology potentially useful for the treatment of certain diseases in the clinics. The success of liposomes as drug carriers has been reflected in a number of liposome-based formulations, which are commercially available or are currently undergoing clinical trials. The current pharmaceutical preparations of liposome-based therapeutic systems mainly result from our understanding of lipid-drug interactions and liposome disposition mechanisms. The insight gained from clinical use of liposome drug delivery systems can now be integrated to design liposomes that can be targeted on tissues, cells or intracellular compartments with or without expression of target recognition molecules on liposome membranes.

Based on their size and number of bilayers liposome's are classified into three basic types:

1) Multilamellar vesicles (MLVs).

2) Small Unilamellar Vesicles (SUVs) and

3) Large Unilamellar Vesicles (LUVs)

Multilamellar vesicles (MLVs). Of several lipid bilayers separated one another by aqueous spaces. They are heterogeneous in size, often ranging from a few hundred to thousands of nanometer in diameter. Both Small Unilamellar Vesicles (SUVs) and Large Unilamellar Vesicles (LUVs) consist of single bilayer surrounding the entrapped aqueous space. SUVs are less than 100nm in size whereas LUVs have diameter larger than 100nm.

In terms of composition and mechanism of intracellular delivery liposomes are classified into five types:

1) Conventional liposomes.

2) pH sensitive liposomes,

3) Cationic liposomes,

4) Immuno liposomes, and

5) Long circulating liposomes.

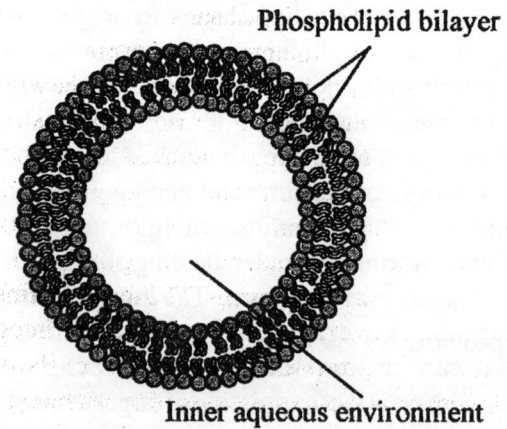

Phospholipid bilayer

Inner aqueous environment

Fig.1: Structure of Liposomes

In order to enchance the activity and to reduce the toxicity of active ingredient a variety of therapeutic and diagnostic agent are delivered through liposomes. Material used in the liposomes formulation depends upon the drug nature. The commonly used material used includes phospholipids, glycophinogolipids, sterols, metabolic fate of bilayer forming lipid, cationic lipid a variety of other lipid and surfactant. Phospholipid bilayer Inner aqueous environment

Advantages of Liposomes

1. Liposomes are biocompatible, completely biodegradable, non-toxic, flexible and nonimmunogenic for systemic and non-systemic administrations.

2. Liposomes supply both a lipophilic environment and aqueous "milieu interne" in one system and are therefore suitable for delivery of hydrophobic, amphipathic and hydrophilic drugs and agents.

3. Liposomes have the ability to protect their encapsulated drug from the external environment and to act as sustained release depots (Propranolol, Cyclosporin).

4. Liposomes can be formulated as a suspension, as an aerosol, or in a semisolid form such as gel, cream and lotion, as a dry vesicular powder (proliposome) for reconstitution or they can be administered through most routes of administration including ocular, pulmonary, nasal, oral, intramuscular, subcutaneous, topical and intravenous, shown in Table 2.

5. Liposomes could encapsulate not only small molecules but also macromolecules like superoxide dismutase, haemoglobin, erythropoietin, interleukin-2 and interferon-g.

6. Liposomes are reduced toxicity and increased stability of entrapped drug via encapsulation. (Amphotericin B, Taxol).

7. Liposomes are increased efficacy and therapeutic index of drug (Actinomycin-D).

8. Liposomes help to reduce exposure of sensitive tissues to toxic drugs.

9. Alter the pharmacokinetic and pharmacodynamic property of drugs (reduced elimination, increased circulation life time).

10. Flexibility to couple with site-specific ligands to achieve active targeting (Anticancer and Antimicrobial drugs).

Disadvantages of liposomes

1. Production cost is high.
2. Leakage and fusion of encapsulated drug / molecules.
3. Sometimes phospholipid undergoes oxidation and hydrolysis like reaction.
4. Short half-life.
5. Low solubility.
6. Fewer stables.

4.2 COMPOSITION OF LIPOSOMES

There are number of the structural and nonstructural components of liposomes, major structural components of liposomes are:

a. Phospholipid

Phospholipid is the major component of the biological membrane; two types of phospholipids are used natural and synthetic phospholipids. The most common natural phospholipid is the phospatidylcholine (PC) is the amphipathic molecule and also known as lecithin. It is originated from animal (hen egg) and vegetable (soyabean).

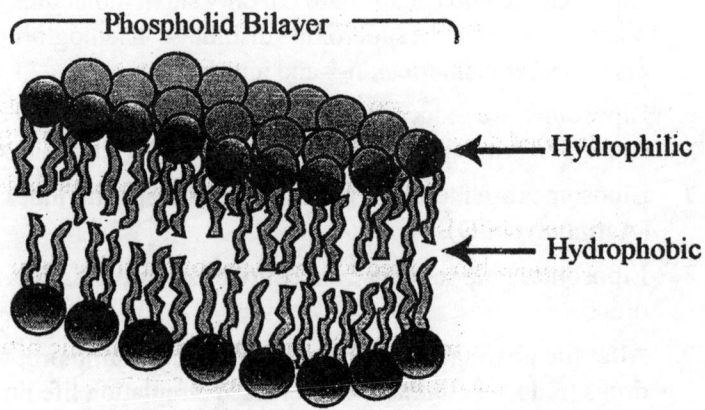

Fig.2: Composition of Phospholipid bilayer

b. Cholesterol

Incorporation of cholesterol in liposome bilayer can bring about big changes in the preparation of these membranes. It does not mean by itself form bilayer membrane structure, but can be incorporated into phospholipids membrane in very high concentration up to 1:1 or 2:1 molar ratios of cholesterol to phospatidylcholine. Being an amphipathic molecule, cholesterol inserts into the membrane with its hydroxyl group of cholesterol oriented towards the aqueous surface and aliphatic chain aligned parallel to the acyl chains in the center of the bilayers and also it increase the separation between choline head groups and eliminates the normal electrostatic and hydrogen bonding interaction.

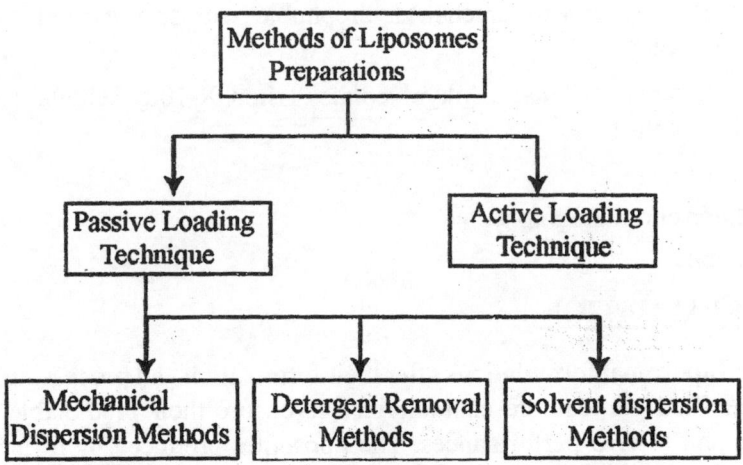

Fig.3: Methods of Liposomes preparations

Mechanical dispersion methods

Lipid is solublised in organic solvent, drug to be entrapped is solubilise in aqueous solvent, the lipid phase is hydrated at high speed stirring due to affinity of aqueous phase to polar head it is entrapped in lipid vesicles.

e.g. Lipid film hydration, Micro-emulsification (Micro fluidizer), Sonication, Dried reconstituted vesicle.

Solvent dispersion methods

In this method, lipids are first dissolved in organic solvent, which then brought in to contact with aqueous phase containing material which is to be entrapped in liposome under rapid dilution and rapid evaporation of organic solvent.

e.g. Ethanol injection, Ether injection, De-emulsification.

Detergent removal method

In this methods, the phospholipids are brought into intimate contact with the aqueous phase via detergent which associate with phospholipids molecules and serve to screen the hydrophobic portions of the molecules from water.

Detergent (Cholate, Alkyglycolate, Triton X-100) removal from mixed micells by

-Dialysis,

-Column chromatography,

-Dilution.

4.3 EVALUATION

Liposomal formulations after their formulation and processing for a specified purpose are characterized to ensure their predictable *in-vitro* and *in-vivo* performances. The liposomes produced by different techniques may have different physicochemical characteristics. These differences may have an impact on their behaviour *in-vivo* (disposition) and *in-vitro*. There are several examples demonstrating the importance of proper selection of liposomes structure to optimize therapeutic effect. The characterization parameters for the purpose of evaluation could be classified into three broad categories, which include:

➢ Physical,

➢ Chemical and

➢ Biological parameters.

Physical characterization evaluates various parameters, including size, shape, surface features, lamellarity, phase behaviour and drug release profile. Chemical characterization includes those studies which establish the purity and potency of various liposomal constituents. Biological characterization parameters are helpful in establishing the safety and suitability of the formulations for the in vivo use or the therapeutic application. Physical and chemical characterizations are very important for meaningful comparison of different liposomes preparations for different batches. Biological consideration helps to ensure safety of use in humans.

Particle size and particle size distribution

The mean particle size and particle size distribution of the optimized batch was obtained by particle size analyzer (Sympatec HELOS, Germany (H1004)). The instrument measures the particle size based on the laser diffraction theory. The apparatus consists of a He-Ne laser beam of 632.8 nm focused with a minimum power of 5 mW using a fourier lens [R-5] to a point at the center of multielement detector and a sample holding unit (Su cell). The sample was stirred using a stirrer before determining the vesicle size. The vesicle dispersions were diluted about 100 times in the deionized water. Diluted liposomal suspension was added to sample dispersion unit containing stirrer and stirred at high speed in order to reduce interparticles aggregation and laser beam was focused.

Drug entrapment efficiency

The liposome suspension was ultra centrifuged at 5000 rpm for 15 minutes at 4°C temperature by using remi cooling centrifuge to separate the free drug. A supernant containing liposomes in suspended stage and free drug at the wall of centrifugation tube. The supernant was collected and again centrifuged at 15000 rpm at 4°C temperature for 30 minutes. A clear solution of supernant and pellets of liposomes were obtained. The pellet containing only liposomes was resuspended in distilled water until further processing. The liposomes free from unentrapped drug were soaked in 10 ml of methanol and then sonicated for 10 min. The vesicles were broken to release the drug, which was then estimated for the drug content. The absorbance of the drug was noted at 222 nm. The entrapment efficiency was then calculated using following equation.

$$100\% \text{ Entrapment efficiency} = \frac{\text{Entrapped Drug}}{\text{Total drug added}} \times 100 \text{ D}$$

In-vitro drug release study from liposomes

Studies of the drug release/diffusion from liposomal system are directed toward the approaches that are relevant to the in vivo condition. *In vitro* diffusion studies were carried out using Franz diffusion cell. Apparatus with a diameter of 25 mm and a diffusional area of 4.90 cm². Regenerated cellulose acetate membrane (thickness of 60–65 im and 0.45 im pore size) was sandwiched between the lower cell reservoir and the glass cell top containing the sample and secured in place with a pinch clamp. The receiving compartment (volume 22 ml) was filled with pH 5 acetate buffer containing 20% v/v methanol (to maintain sink condition). The system was maintained at 37±0.5 °C by magnetic heater, resulting in a membrane-surface temperature of 32 °C . A Teflon TM coated magnetic bar continuously stirred the receiving medium to avoid diffusion layer effects. A sample was placed evenly on the surface of the membrane in the donor compartment. 2 ml of receptor fluid were withdrawn from the receiving compartment at 1, 2, 3, 4, 6, 8, 10 & 12 hours and replaced with 2 ml of fresh solution. Samples were assayed spectrophotometrically for drug content.

Therapeutic applications of liposomes

1.   Liposomes as drug / protein delivery vehicles

   ➤ Controlled and sustain release *in situ*

   ➤ Enhanced drug solubilization

   ➤ Enzyme replacement therapy and lysosomal storage disorders

   ➤ Altered pharmacokinetics and biodistribution

2.   Liposomes in antimicrobial, antifungal and antiviral therapy

3.   Liposomes in tumour therapy

   ➤ Carrier of small cytotoxic molecules.

   ➤ Vehicle for macromolecules as cytokines and genes.

4.   Liposomes in gene delivery

➢ Genes and Antisense therapy.

➢ Genetic (DNA) vaccination.

5. Liposomes in immunology.

6. Liposomes as radiopharmaceutical and radio diagnostic carrier.

7. Liposomes in cosmetic and dermatology.

8. Liposomes in enzyme immobilization and bioreactor technology.

Table1: Therapeutic applications of liposomes

Drug	Route of Administration	Application	Targeted Diseases
Amphotericin-B	Oral delivery	Ergosterol membrane	Mycotic infection
Insulin	Oral, Ocular Pulmonary and Transderaml delivery	Decrease Glucose level	Diabetic mellitus
Ketoprofen	Ocular delivery	Cyclo-Oxygenase enzyme inhibitor	Pain muscle condition
Pentoxyfylline	Pulmonary delivery	Phosphodiesterase	Asthma
Tobramycin	Pulmonary delivery	Protein synthesis inhibitor	Pseudomonas infection acruginosa
Salbutamol	Pulmonary delivery	β_2- adrenorecoptor antagonist	Asthma
Cytarabin	Pulmonary delivery	DNA-Polymerase inhibition	Acute-leukemias
Benzocain	Transdermal	Inhibition of nerve impulse from sensory nerves	Ulcer on mucous suface with pain
Ketoconazole	Transdermal	Inhibit ergosterol	Candida-albican's

4.4 NANOPARTICLES

Nanoparticles are defined as particulate dispersions or solid particles with a size in the range of 10-1000nm. The drug is dissolved, entrapped, encapsulated or attached to a nanoparticle matrix. Depending upon the method of preparation, nanoparticles, nanospheres or nanocapsules can be obtained. Nanocapsules are systems in which the drug is confined to a cavity surrounded by a unique polymer membrane, while nanospheres are matrix systems in which the drug is physically and uniformly dispersed. In recent years, biodegradable polymeric nanoparticles, particularly those coated with hydrophilic polymer such as poly(ethylene glycol) (PEG) known as long-circulating particles, have been used as potential drug delivery devices because of their ability to circulate for a prolonged period time target a particular organ, as carriers of DNA in gene therapy, and their ability to deliver proteins, peptides and genes. The major goals in designing nanoparticles as a delivery system are to control particle size, surface properties and release of pharmacologically active agents in order to achieve the site-specific action of the drug at the therapeutically optimal rate and dose regimen. Though liposomes have been used as potentialcarriers with unique advantages including protecting drugs from degradation, targeting to site of action and reduction toxicity or side effects, their applications are limited due to inherent problems such as low encapsulation efficiency, rapid leakage of water-soluble drug in the presence of blood components and poor storage stability. On the other hand, polymeric nanoparticles offer some specific advantages over liposomes. For instance, they help to increase the stability of drugs/proteins and possess useful controlled release properties.

Types Of Nanoparticles

1. Quantum Dots

2. Nanocrystalline Silicon

3. Photonic

4. Crystals

5. Liposome

6. Gliadin Nanoparticles

7. Polymeric Nanoparticles

8. Solid Lipid Quantum Nanoparticles (SLN)

Others-gold,carbon,silver,etc.

POLYMERS USED IN THE PREPARATION OF NANOPARTICLES:

I)Natural hydrophilic polymers

A)Proteins:

➢ Gelatin

➢ Albumin

➢ Lectin

B)Polysaccharides:

➢ Alginate

➢ Dextran

➢ Chitosan

➢ Agarose

Nanospheres: Solid core spherical particulate which are nanometric in size.

Nanocapsules: Are vesicular system with drug is essentially encapsulated within

embryonic polymer sheath.

Nanocrystals: Drug is mainly encapsulated within the solution system.

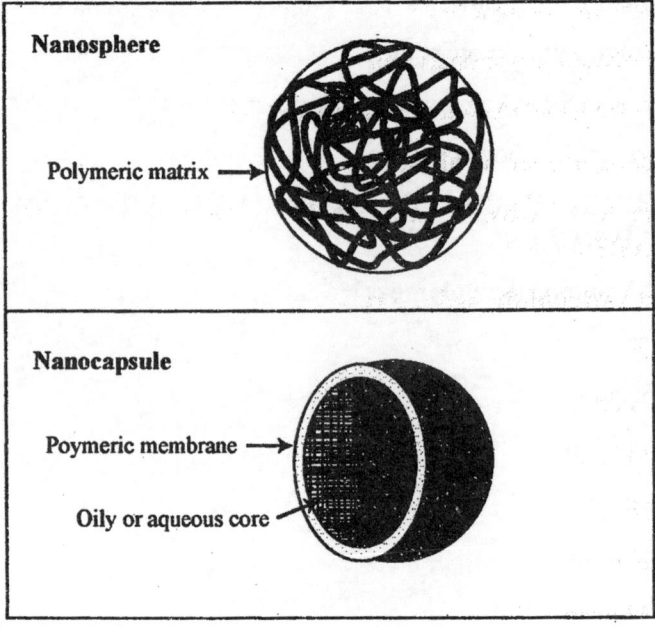

Fig.4: Nanoparticles

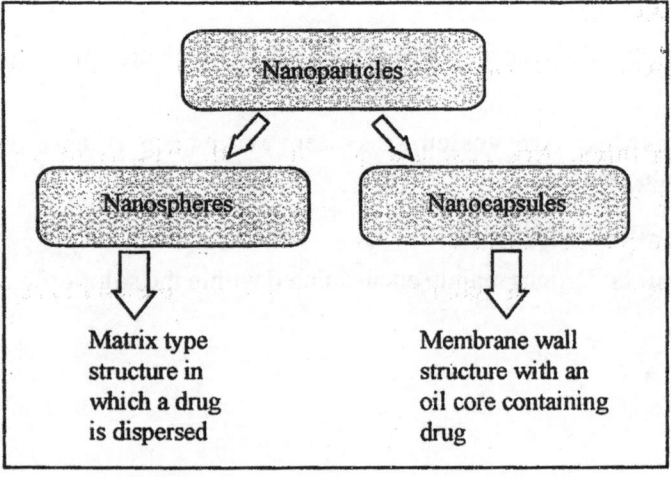

Fig.5: Preparation techniques

II) Synthetic hydrophobic polymers:

A) Pre polymerized

➢ Poly(E-caprolactone)-PECL.

➢ Poly(lactic acid)-PLA.

➢ Poly(lactide-co-glycolide)-PLGA.

➢ Polystyrene.

B)Polymerized in process

➢ Poly(isobutyl cyanoacryaltes)-PICA

➢ Poly(butylcyanoacrylate)-PBCA

➢ Poly(hexyl cyanoacrylate)-PHCA

➢ Poly(methyl methacrylate)-PMMA

4.5 PREPARATION TECHNIQUES OF NANOPARTICLES

The selection of the appropriate method for the preparation of nanoparticles depends on the physic chemical characteristics of the polymer and the drug to be loaded.

The preparation techniques largely determine the minor structure,invitro release profile and the biological fate of these polymeric delivery systems.

Two types of systems with different inner structures are possible.

i) A matrix type systems consisting of an entanglement of oligomer or polymer units(nanoparticles/spheres

ii)A reservoir type of system consisting of oily core surrounded by an embryonic polymeric shell.(nanocapsules)

The methods of preparation of nanaoparticles are classified as

1) Amphiphilic macromolecule crossly linking

a) Heat cross linking

b) Chemical cross linking

2) Polymerization based methods

a) Polymerization of monomers insitu

b) Emulsion(micellar)polymerization

c) Dispersion polymerization

d) Interfacial condensation polymerization

e) Interfacial complexation

3) Polymer precipitation methods

a) Solvent extraction/evaporation

b) Solvent displacement (nanoprecipitation)

c) Salting Out

1) Amphiphilic Macromolecule crosslinking

➤ Nanoparticles can be prepared from amphilic macromolecules,proteins and polysaccharides which have affinity for aqueous and lipid solvents.

➤ The technique involves firstly the aggregation of amphiphiles followed by further stabilization either by heat denaturation or chemical cross linking.

a) Heat crosslinking

The method involves the emulsification of bovine serum albumin or human serum albumin or protein aqueous solution in oil using high pressure homogenization or high frequency sonication.

The water in oil emulsion so formed is then poured into preheated oil.(temperature above 100c)

The suspension in pre heated oil maintained above 100c is held stirred for a specific period of time in order to denaturate and aggregate -the protein contents of aqueous pool completely and to evaporate the water.

The particles formed are finally washed with an organic solvent to remove any adherent or adsorbed oil traces and subsequently collected by centrifugation.

b) Chemical cross linking

The high temperature used in the previous method restricts the application of method to temperature sensitive drugs.

As an alternative,a chemical cross linking agent usually glutaraldehyde is incorporated into the system at a concentration of 3%v/v.

II) Polymerization based methods

a) Two different approaches are generally adopted for the preparation of nanospheres using insitu polymerization technique.

➤ Emulsion polymerization,in which the monomer to be polymerized is emulsified in a non solvent phase.

➤ Dispersion polymerization in which the monomer is dissolved in a solvent that is non solvent for the resulting polymer.

In emulsion polymerization,the monomer is dissolved in an internal phase while in case of dispersion polymerization ,it is taken in dispersed phase.

b) Emulsion polymerization

Two different mechanisms were proposed for the emulsion polymerization process.

i)Micellar nucleation and polymerization

ii)Homogenous nucleation and polymerization

i) Micellar nucleation and polymerization:

It involves the swollen monomer micelles as the site of nucleation and polymerization.

The monomer is emulsified in the nonsolvent phase with the help of surfactant molecules.

The process leads to the formation of monomer swollen micelles and stabilized monomer droplets. The polymerization reaction proceeds through nucleation and propagation stage in the presence of a chemical or physical initiator. The energy provided by the initiator creates free reactive monomers in the continuous phase, which then collide with surrounding unreactive monomers and initiate the polymerization chain reaction. Being slightly soluble iun the surrounding phase,the monomer molecules reach the micelles by diffusion from the monomer droplets through the continuous phase,thus allowing the polymerization to progress within the micelles. Poly (alkyl cyanoacrylate),biodegradable,polymer.

ii) Homogenous nucleation and polymerization

In this case monmer is sufficiently soluble in the continuous outer phase. The nucleation and polymorphism stages can directly occur in this phase,leading to the formation of primary chains called oligomers. When the oligomers have reached a certain length,they precipitate and form primary particles, which are stablized by the surfactant molecules provided by the micelles and the droplets.

c) Dispersion polymerization

Here the monomer is dissolved in an aqueous medium which acts as a precipitant for subsequently formed polymer. The monomer is introduced into the dispersion medium of an emulsion or an inversed emulsion into non solvent based polymeric solution. The nucleation solution is directly induced in the aqueous monomer solution and the presence of stabilizer or surfactants is not absolutely necessary for the formation of stable nanospheres. This method is used to prepare biodegradable polyacrylamide & PMMA nanoparticles. Subsequently completing poly electrolyte is added to the bulk,which causes a layer of insoluble poly electrolyte complex to coacervate at the interface.

d) Interfacial polymerization

In this method,the preformed polymer phase is finally transformed to an embryonic sheath. A polymer that eventually becomes core of nanoparticles and drug molecules to be loaded are dissolve in a volatile solvent. The solution is then poured into a non solvent for both polymer and core phase. The polymer phase is separated as a coacervative phase at o/w interface. The resultant mixture instantaneously turns milky owing to the formation of nanocapsules. Then size of the nanocapsules ranges from 30-300nm and the drug loading efficiency critically depends on drug solubility in core phase. Interfacial polymerization for the encapsulation of proteins, enzymes, antibodies and cells was employed and extensively used.

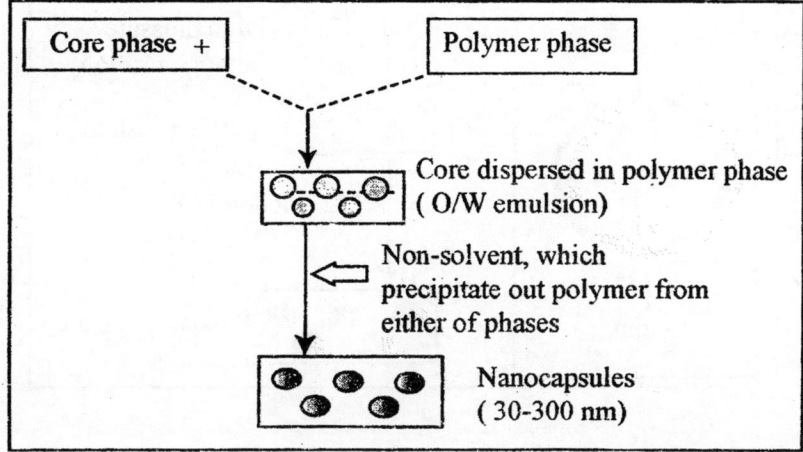

Fig.6: Preparation of nanoparticles by interfacial polymerization

e) Interfacial complexation

The method is based on the process of microencapsulation. In the case of nanoparticle preparation, aqueous polyelectrolyte solution is carefully dissolved in reverse micelles in an a polar bulk phase with the help of an appropriate surface active agent.

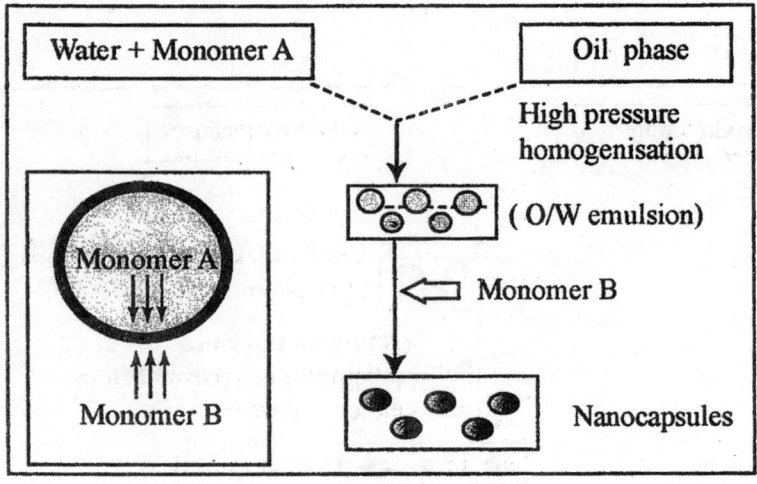

Fig.7: Preparation of nanoparticles by interfacial complexation.

3) Polymer precipitation methods

In these methods, the hydrophobic polymer and/ or a hydrophobic drug is dissolved in a particular organic solvent follwed by its dispersion in a continuous aqueous phase in which the polymer is insoluble.

The polymer precipitation occurs as a consequence of the sovent extraction or evaporation, which can be brought about by:

➤ Increasing the solubility of the organic solvent in the external medium by adding an alcohol.

➤ By incorporating additional amount of water into the ultra emulsion (to extract/diffuse the solvent).

➤ By evaporation of the organic solvent at room temperature or at accelerated temperature or by using vacuum.

➤ Using the organic solvent that is completely soluble in the continuous phase. (Ex: acetone). Nanoprecipitation.

a) Solvent extraction method

This method involves the formation of a conventional o/w emulsion between a partially water miscible solvent containing the polymer and the drug and an aqueous phase containing the stabilizer. The subsequent removal of the solvent(solvent evaporation) or the addition water to the system so as to affect diffusion of the solvent to the external phase (emulsification diffusion) are the two variance of the solvent extraction method. Sonication, high speed/pressure homogenization methods are widely employed for evaporation. Recently emulsification-diffusion method has been used for the solvent extraction process.

a) Double emulsion solvent evaporation method

Emulsion solvent evaporation technique has been further modified and a double emulsion(or multiple emulsion) of water in oil in water type has been used. Drug along with polymer is dissolved in organic solvent and stabilizer is added to water separately.

These two solutions are mixed and sonicated or homogenized to form w/o emulsion.

This emulsion is further added to a PVA aqueous solution to yield the water in oil in water double emulsion. The organic solvent is allowed to evaporate. Following the evaporation of the organic solvents/ nanoparticles are formed which are then recovered by ultra centrifugation, washed repetitively with buffer and lyophilized.

b) Solvent displacement or nanoprecipitation:

This method involves the use of an organic phase, which is completely soluble in the external aqueous phase.

The organic solvent diffuses instantaneously to the external aqueous phase, including immediate polymer precipitation because of the complete miscibility of the both phases.

After nanoparticle preparation, the solvent is eliminated and the free flowing nanoparticles can be obtained under reduced pressure.

This method is particularly useful for drugs that are slightly soluble in water. If the drug is highly hydrophilic, it diffuses out into the external aqueous phase, where as if the drug highly hydrophobic, it may precipitate in the aqueous phase as nanocrystals, which further grow during storage.

In case hydrophilic polymer, an aqueous solution of polymer is dispersed or emulsified in oil phase. The precipitaion of polymer proceeds on addition of acetone.

d)Salting out

This method involves the incorporation of a saturated aqueous solution of PVA into an acetone solution of the polymer undern magnetic stirring to form an O/W emulsion. The precipitation of the polymer occurs when a sufficient amount of water is added to external phase to allow complete diffusion of the acetone from internal phase into the aqueous phase. This technique is suitable for drugs and polymers that are soluble in polar solvents, such as acetone or ethanol.

4.6 APPLICATIONS

➢ Intracellular targeting of anti-infective drugs

➢ Specific targeting of anti-inflammatory drugs to areas of inflammation.

➢ In ocular delivery to deliver pilocarpine and other miotic drugs.

➢ As carriers for radio nucleotides for diagnostic purposes in nuclear medicine.

➢ To improve the solubility and bioavailability of poorly soluble drugs.

➢ For skin and hair care in the form of solid lipid nanoparticles.

➢ To deliver the drugs across the Blood brain barrier (BBB).

➢ To formulate sustained release formulations.

➢ For targeted delivery of proteins and peptides.

➢ As adjuvants to render antigens potent enough to be useful for vaccines.

Table 2: Evaluation Parameter of Nano particle

Parameters	Characterization methods
Particle size & size distribution	Photon correlation spectroscopy, Scanning electron microscopy(SEM), Transmission eletron microscopy(TEM), Atomic force microscopy(AFM), Mercury porository,
Charge determination	Laser droplet Anemometry, Zeta potentiometer
Surface hydrophobicity	Water contact angle measurements, Rose bangle (dye) binding, hydrophobic interaction chromatography, X-Ray photoeletron spectroscopy
Chemical analysis of surface	Static secondary ion mass spectroscopy, sorptometer
Carrier drug interaction	Differential scanning calorimetry
Nanoparticle dispersion stability	Critical flocculation temparature (CFT)
Release profile	*In Vitro* release characteristic under physiologic & sink condition
Drug stability	Bioassay of drug extracted from nanoparticle, Chemical analysis of drug.

Parameter which are to be evaluated:

➤ Particle size,

➤ Zeta potential,

➤ Drug release,

➤ Surface morphology.

➤ Polymorphism,

➤ Degree of crystallinity,

➤ Time scale of distribution processes.

Particle size and Zeta potential

There are so many techniques for the particle size and zeta potential (size distribution) like photon correlation spectroscopy (PCS), transmission electron microscopy (TEM), scanning electron microscopy (SEM), atomic force microscopy (AFM), scanning tunneling microscopy (STM) or freeze fracture electron microscopy (FFEM). For the routine measurement of particle size.Photon correlation spectroscopy (PCS) and laser diffraction (LD) are important techniques used. Coulter counter are rarely used to measure particle size because of difficulties in the assessment of small nanoparticle. Photon correlation spectroscopy (PCS) is not able to detect larger microparticles. Difficulties may arise both in PCS and LD measurements for samples which contain several populations of different size. Therefore, additional techniques might be useful like light microscopy it gives fast indication of the presence and character of microparticles. Electron microscopy provides, in contrast to PCS and LD, direct information on the particle shape. However, the investigator should pay special attention to possible artifacts which may be caused by the sample preparation. For example, solvent removal may cause modifications which will influence the particle shape. Zeta potential is an important product characteristic of SLNs since its high value is expected to lead to deaggregation of particles in the absence of other complicating factors such as steric stabilizers or hydrophilic surface appendages. It is usually measured by zetameter.

Drug content

Drug content is determined by centrifugation method. The redispersed nanoparticles suspension is centrifuged at 15,000 rpm for 40 min at 25° to separate the free drug in the supernatant. Concentration in the supernatant is determined by UV-Vis spectrophotometyrically at 271 nm after suitable dilution.

Electron microscopy

Scanning electron microscopy (SEM) and transmission electron microscopy (TEM) provide a way to directly observe nanoparticles and physical characterization of nanoparticles. TEM has a smaller size limit of detection, is a good validation for other methods and one must be cognizant of the statistically small sample size and the effect that vacuum can have on the particles.

Nuclear Magnetic Resonance (NMR)

NMR is used to determine both size and nature of nanoparticles. The selectivity afforded by chemical shift complements the sensitivity to molecular mobility to provide information on the physicochemical status of components within the nanoparticle.

X-Ray Diffraction And Differential Scanning Calorimetry (DSC)

The geometric scattering of radiation from crystal planes within a solid allow the presence or absence of the former to be determined thus permitting the degree of crystallinity to be assessed. DSC can be used to determine the nature and speciation of crystallinity within nanoparticles through the measurement of glass and melting point temperatures and their associated enthalpies.

Atomic Force Microscopy (AFM)

In this technique, a probe tip with atomic scale sharpness is kept across a sample to produce a topological map based on the forces at play between the tip and the surface. The probe can be dragged across the sample (contact mode) or allowed to hover just above (noncontact mode), with the exact nature of the particular force employed serving to distinguish among the sub techniques. That ultrahigh resolution is obtainable with this approach, which along with the ability to map a sample according to properties in addition to size.

In vitro release studies

In vitro release studies is carried out by using dialysis tubes with an artificial membrane. The prepared nanoparticles and 10 ml of phosphate buffer is added to the dialysis tube and subjected to dialysis by immersing the dialysis tube to the receptor compartment containing 250 ml of phosphate buffer. The medium in the receptor is agitated continuously using a magnetic stirrer a temperature is maintained at $37\pm1°$. 5ml of sample of receptor compartment is taken at various intervals of time over a period of 24 h and each time fresh buffer is replaced. The amount of drug released is determined spectrometrically.

4.7 RESEALED ERYTHROCYTES

INTRODUCTION

Erythrocytes, also known as red blood cells, have been extensively studied for their potential carrier capabilities for the delivery of drugs and drug-loaded microspheres. Such drug-loaded *carrier erythrocytes* are prepared simply by collecting blood samples from the organism of interest, separating erythrocytes from plasma, entrapping drug in the erythrocytes, and resealing the resultant cellular carriers. Hence, these carriers are called *resealed erythrocytes*. The overall process is based on the response of these cells under osmotic conditions. Upon reinjection, the drug-loaded erythrocytes serve as slow circulating depots and target the drugs to a reticuloendothelial system (RES).

The developing RBC has the capacity to synthesize hemoglobin. But the adult erythrocytes lose this capacity and serve only to carry hemoglobin. The membrane mainly encloses cytoplasm and a red pigment called hemoglobin. The cells on resealing lose some of the properties of normal erythrocytes and referred as "Resealed Erythrocytes" such erythrocytes which contain no or little hemoglobin are called ghosts.

Morphology and physiology of erythrocytes

Erythrocytes are the most abundant cells in the human body (~5.4 million cells/mm3 blood in a healthy male and ~4.8 million cells/mm3 blood in a healthy female). These cells were described in human blood samples by Dutch Scientist Lee Van Hock in 1674. In the 19th century, Hope Seyler identified hemoglobin and its crucial role in oxygen delivery to various parts of the body . Erythrocytes are biconcave discs with an average diameter of 7.8 µm, a thickness of 2.5 µm in periphery, 1 µm in the center, and a volume of 85–91 µm3. The flexible, biconcave shape enables erythrocytes to squeeze through narrow capillaries, which may be only 3 µm wide. Mature erythrocytes are quite simple in structure. They lack a nucleus and other organelles. Their plasma membrane encloses hemoglobin, a heme-containing protein that is responsible for O_2–CO_2 binding inside the erythrocytes. The main role of erythrocytes is the transport of O_2 from the lungs to tissues and the CO_2 produced in tissues back to lungs. Thus, erythrocytes are a highly specialized O_2

carrier system in the body. Because a nucleus is absent, all the intracellular space is available for O2 transport. Also, because mitochondria are absent and because energy is generated anaerobically in erythrocytes, these cells do not consume any of the oxygen they are carrying. Erythrocytes live only about 120 days because of wear and tear on their plasma membranes as they squeeze through the narrow blood capillaries. Worn-out erythrocytes are removed from circulation and destroyed in the spleen and liver (RES), and the breakdown products are recycled. The process of erythrocyte formation within the body is known as *erythropoiesis*. In a mature human being, erythrocytes are produced in red bone marrow under the regulation of a hemopoietic hormone called *erythropoietin.*

Advantages

➢   Biodegradable in nature.

➢   Isolation of erythrocytes is easy.

➢   Larger amount of drug can be encapsulated in a small volume of cells

➢   Non-immunogenic in action.

➢   Prolong the systemic activity of the drug while residing for a longer time in the body.

➢   Prolong the systemic activity of the drug while residing for a longer time in the body.

➢   They can target the drug with (reticuloendothelial system)RES.

Disadvantages

➢   They have a limited potential as carrier to non-phagocytic tissue.

➢   Possibility of clumping of cells and dose dumping.

Requirments for encapsulatioin

➢   A wide variety of biologically active substances can be entrapped in erythorcytes.

➢   Generally, the molecules should be polar or hydrophilic.

➢   Once encapsulated, charged molecules are retained longer than uncharged molecule.

➢   The hydrophobic molecules can be entrapped in erythrocytes by absorbing over other molecules.

Ex:-Adriamycin was entrapped in human erythrocytes in their respective salts.

Ex:-Tetracycline hydrocholoride salt can be appreciably entrapped in bovine RBC.

4.8 ISOLATION OF ERYTHROCYTES

The cellular content is about 45% of the blood volume and contains

1) Erythrocytes(RBC)

2) Leuckocytes(WBC) and

3) Thrombocytes (Platelets).

➢ The plasma is primarily water (90 to 92%) & protein (7%).

➢ Blood is withdrawn from cardiac/splenic puncture (in case of small animals) and through veins (in case of large animals) in to a syringe containing a drop of anticoagulant.The whole blood is centrifuged at 2500 rpm for 5min at 4±1°c in a refrigerated centrifuge.

➢ The serum and buffy coats are carefully removed and packed cells were washed 3 times with phosphate buffer saline (PH 7.4).

➢ The washed erythrocytes are stored at 4°C until used.

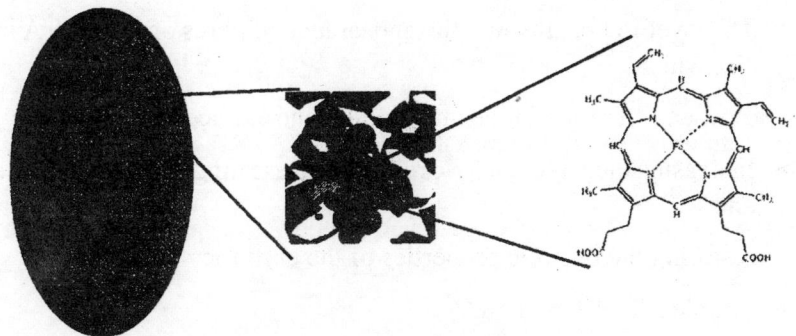

Fig.8: Composition Of Erthrocyte.

Entrapment Methods

1) Hypo-Osmotic lysis method.

    a) Dilution Method

    b) Dialysis Method

    c) Preswell Method

    d) Isotonic Osmotic Lysis Method.

2) Electrical breakdown Method.

3) Endocytosis Method.

4) Membrane perturbation method.

5) Normal transport method.

6) Lipid is fusion method.

7) Hypo-osmotic lysis method.

Dilution Method

➤ In this method the RBC are exposed to hypotonic conditions (0.4% Nacl), where water will enter and will swell the cell.

➢ The cell swells upto 1.6 times its original volume.

➢ The swelling results into the appearance of pores of 200-500 A in size which

allow equilibration of the intracellular and extracellular volume.

➢ Increasing the ionic stat 37^0c results into resealing of cell membrane and

restoring the osmotic properties of the erythrocytes.

➢ Simple and fast method.

➢ Efficient for encapsulation of low molecular weight drugs.

Disadvantages

➢ Encapsulation efficiency is very low i.e. 1 to 8%.

Dialysis Method

➢ A desired hematocrit is achieved by mixing erythrocyte suspension and drug solution.

➢ This mixture is placed into a dialysis tubing and then both ends of the tube are tied with thread.

➢ In air bubble of nearly 25% of the internal volume is put in the tube.

➢ The bottle is placed at 4°c for the desired lysistime.

➢ The contents of the dialysis tube are mixed by shaking the tube.

➢ The dia ysis tube is then placed in 100ml of resealing solution. (isotonic, PBS, PH 7.4) at room temperature.

➢ The loaded erythrocytes thus obtained are then washed with cold PBS at 4°c.

➢ The cells are finally resuspended in the PBS.

Preswell Dilution Technique

➢ The erythrocytes are allowed to swell without lysis by placing then in slightly hypotonic solution.

➢ The swollen cells are recovered by centrifugation at low speed.

➢ Then, relatively small volumes of aqueous drug solution are added to the point of lysis.

➢ This method is simpler and quicker and produces erythrocytes carriers which have good in vivo survival.

Isotonic Osmotic Lysis Technique

➢ In this method, RBC are suspended in propylene glycol which causes a transient-permeability in RBC wall which allows drugs and other agents to diffuse in.

➢ The lysed erythrocytes are resealed under isotonic condition by dilution with a glycol free medium.

Electrical Breakdown Method

➢ This method follows electrical haemolysis.

➢ In the presence of high electric field of approx 104 volts/cm for a period of <50 sec. The RBC membrane experiences a dielectric break down followed by ion leakage and haemolysis.

➢ Stable pores are formed in the membrane allowing entrapment of drug molecules.

Endocytosis

➢ Intracellular vesicles could be induced in erythrocytes containing small molecules drug from external medium.

➢ In this methd, the vesicle membrane seperate the endocytosed substance from the cytoplasm containing drug, which are sensitive to inactivation by cytoplasmic enzyme and also protect the erythrocyte membrane.

Membrane Perturbation

➢ Antibiotics such as amphotericin-â damage micro-organisms by increasing the permeability of their membrane to metabolites and ions.

➢ This properly can be utilized for loading of drug into erythrocytes.

Ex:-Amphotericin-â was used to load erythrocytes with antileukaemic drug daunomycin.

Normal Transport Mechanism

➢ It is possible to load erythrocytes with drug without disrupting the erythrocyte membrane.

➢ Here, the drug and erythrocytes are together incubated for a varying period of time.

Characterization

1) Drug contents

2) In-vitro drug release

3) Percent cell recovery.

4) Morphology.

5) Osmotic fragility.

6) Osmotic shock

7) Turbulence shock.

8) Erythrocyte sedimentation rate.

9) Zeta sedimentation rate.

Parameter	Method/Instrument used
I. Physical characterization	
Shape and surface morphology	Transmission electron microscopy, Scanning electron microscopy, Phase contrast microscopy, Optical microscopy
Vesicle size and size distribution	Transmission electron microscopy, Optical microscopy
Drug release	Diffusion cell, dialysis
Drug content	Deproteinization of cell membrane followed by assay of resealed drug, radaiolabelling
Surface electrical potential	Zeta potential measurement
Surface pH	pH- sensitive probles
Deformability	Capillary method
11. Cellular Characterization	
% Hb content	Deproteinization of cellmembrane followed by hemoglobin assay
Cell volume	Laser light scattering
% Cell recovery	Neubaur's chamber, hemotalogical analyser
Osmotic fragility	Stepwise incubation with isotonic to hypotonic sanile solutionsand determination of drug and hemoglobin assay
Osmotic Shock	Dilution with distilled water and estimation of drug hemoglobin
Turbulent shock	Passage of cell suspension through 30-gauge hypedermic needle at 10ml/min flow rate and estomation of residual drug and hemoglobin, vigorous shaking followed by hemoglobin estimation
Erythrocyte sedimentation rate	ESR methods

Applications

➤ Targeting of bioactive agents to reticuloendothelial system (RES).

➤ Treatment of lysosomal storage disease.

➤ Treatment of liver tumors.

➤ Treatment of parasitic diseases.

➤ Removal of RES iron overload.

➤ Targeting of mycotoxins to reticuloendothelial system (RES).

➤ As circulating carriers.

➤ As circulatin bioreactors

➤ In enzyme delivery.

➤ Prevention of thromboembolism.

REVIEW QUESTIONS

ESSAY QUESTIONS

1. What are targeted drug delivery systems? Explain different types of targeted drug delivery systems and their limitations?

2. a. What are liposomes. Write a note on their structure and composition?

   b. Explain their stabilization techniques.

3. Write about classification and characterization of liposomes?

4. What are various approaches for the preparation of liposomes?

5. Write the preparation and characterization techniques of Resealed erythrocytes?

6. Write the routes of administration, storage mechanism of release of Resealed erythrocytes?

7. What are nanoparticles . How nanoparticles are differ from microspheres . Discuss structure , production and various evaluation method for nanoparticles?

SHORT QUESTIONS

1. Write the applications of
   a) Resealed erythrocytes
   b) liposomes
   c) nanoparticles
2. Briefly explain the evaluation of liposome.

Chapter 5

INTRODUCTION TO DRUG REGULATORY AGENCIES

5.1 INTRODUCTION

INDIAN CENTRAL DRUGS STANDARD CONTROL ORGANIZATION (CDSCO)

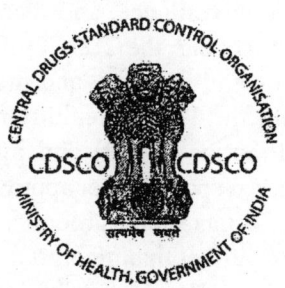

The **Central Drug Standards Control Organization (CDSCO)** regulates drugs, cosmetics, diagnostics and devices in India. It is headed by the **Drug Controller General of India (DCGI)** , responsible for the safety, efficacy, and quality standards for pharmaceuticals and medical devices, and publishes the Indian Pharmacopoeia. The DCGI is advised by the **Drug Technical Advisory Board (DTAB)** and the **Drug Consultative Commission (DCC)**. All licenses for medical devices are handled by the **Central Licensing Approval Authority (CLAA)**. State governments are responsible for licensing, approvals, inspection and recalls of drugs manufactured within their domain. India's main regulatory body for pharmaceuticals and medical devices. Within the CDSCO, the Drug Controller General of

India (DCGI) is responsible for the regulation of pharmaceuticals and medical devices. The DCGI is advised by the Drug Technical Advisory Board (DTAB) and the Drug Consultative Committee (DCC). Licensing and classification of medical devices are handled by the Central Licensing Approval Authority (CLAA). The CLAA is also responsible for setting and enforcing safety standards, appointing notified bodies to oversee conformity assessment, conducting post-market surveillance and issuing warnings and recalls for adverse events.

The CDSCO establishes safety, efficacy, and quality standards for pharmaceuticals and medical devices. It publishes and updates the Indian Pharmacopeia, a list of regulated pharmaceuticals and devices. For all drug and device applications, the CDSCO appoints notified bodies to perform conformity assessment procedures, including testing, in order to ensure compliance with their standards. The CDSCO is also divided into several zonal offices which do pre-licensing and post-licensing inspections, post-market surveillance, and recalls when necessary. In addition to its regulatory functions, the CDSCO offers technical guidance, trains regulatory officials and analysts, and monitors adverse events. The CDSCO works with the World Health Organization to promote Good Manufacturing Practice (GMP) and international regulatory harmony. This organization responsible for approval / issuance of licenses for various categories of drugs such as blood and blood products, I.V. Fluids, vaccines, sera etc., either manufactured in India or imported. It regulates the manufacturing, sale and distribution of drugs through State Authorities and registers the manufactures, suppliers and importers for new drugs, clinical trials etc. It has four zonal offices at Kolkata, Mumbai, Chennai and Ghaziabad which work in close collaboration with State Drug Control Organizations.

5.2 CENTRAL DRUGS STANDARD CONTROL ORGANIZATION

(a) Central Authorities

Under the Drug and Cosmetics Act, the regulation of manufacture, sale and distribution of Drugs is primarily the concern of the State authorities while the Central Authorities are responsible for approval of New Drugs, Clinical Trials in the country, laying down the standards for

Drugs, control over the quality of imported Drugs, coordination of the activities of State Drug Control Organisations and providing expert advice with a view of bring about the uniformity in the enforcement of the Drugs and Cosmetics Act.

Drug Controller General of India is responsible for approval of licenses of specified categories of Drugs such as blood and blood products, I. V. Fluids, Vaccine and Sera.

Central Drugs Standard Control Organization Head quarter is located at FDA Bhawan, Kotla Road, New Delhi 110002 and functions under the Directorate General of Health Services.

Central Drugs Standard Control Organization Head quarter is located at FDA Bhawan, Kotla Road, New Delhi 110002 and functions under the Directorate General of Health Services.

ZONAL OFFICES OF CENTRAL DRUGS STANDARD CONTROL ORGANISATION (CDSCO)

The Central Government have established four zonal offices of the Central Drug Standard Control Organisation at Mumbai, Kolkata, Chennai, and Ghaziabad. The Zonal Offices work in close collabration with the State Drug Control Administration and assist them in securing uniform enforcement of the Drug Act and other connected legislations, on all India basis. The names of the office-in-charge of the Zonal Organisations, their address and names of the States are as follows:

EAST ZONE

Andaman and Nicobar Island, Arunachal Pradesh, Assam, Bihar, Jharkhand, Manipur, Meghalaya, Mizoram, Nagaland, Orissa, Sikkim, Tripura & West Bengal.

WEST ZONE

Chattisgarh, Goa, Daman & Diu, Gujarat, Madhya Pradesh and Maharashtra

NORTH ZONE

Haryana, Himachal Pradesh, Jammu & Kashmir, Punjab, Rajasthan, Uttaranchal, Uttar Pradesh, N.C.T. of Delhi & Union Territory of Chandigarh

SOUTH ZONE

Andhra Pradesh, Karnataka, Kerala, Pondicherry and Tamil Nadu.

Central Drugs Laboratory (CDL)

The Central Drugs Laboratory, Kolkata is the national statutory laboratory of the Government of India for quality control of Drug and Cosmetics and is established under the Indian Drug & Cosmetics Act, 1940. It is the oldest quality control laboratory of the Drug Control Authorities in India. It functions under the administrative control of the Director-General of Health Services in the Ministry of Health and Family Welfare.

The functions of the Laboratory include:

I. Statutory Functions:

(a) Analytical quality control of majority of the imported Drug available in Indian market.

(b) Analytical quality control of drug and cosmetics manufactured within the country on behalf of the Central and State Drug Controller Administrations.

(c) Acting as an Appellate authority in matters of disputes relating to quality of Drug.

II. Other Functions:

i) Collection, storage and distribution of International Standard International Referenc Preparations of Drug and Pharmaceutical Substances.

ii) Preparation of National Reference Standards and maintenance of such Standards. Maintenance of microbial cultures useful in drug analysis Distribution of Standards and cultures to State Quality Control Laboratories and drug manufacturing establishments.

iii) Training of Drug Analysts deputed by State Drug Control Laboratories and other Institutions.

iv) Training of World Health Organisation Fellows from abroad on modern methods of Drug Analysis.

v) To advise the Central Drug Control Administration in respect of quality and toxicity of drug awaiting licence.

vi) To work out analytical specifications for preparation of Monographs for the Indian Pharmacopoeia and the Homoeopathic Pharmacopoeia of India.

vii) To undertake analytical research on standardisation and methodology of Drug and cosmetics.

viii) Analysis of Cosmetics received as survey samples from Central Drug Standard Control Organisation.

ix) Quick analysis of life saving Drug on an All-India basis received under National Survey of Quality of Essential Drug Programme from Zonal Offices of Central Drug Standard Control Organisation.

In addition to the above functions the Central Drug Laboratory also actively collaborates with the World Health Organisation in the preparation of International Standards and Specifications for International Pharmacopoeia. It also undertakes collaborative study on behalf of the Indian Pharmacopoeia Committee. The senior Officers of the Laboratory have been appointed as Government Analysts on behalf of most of the States of the Union for analysis of drug samples.

Regional Drugs Testing Laboratory (RDTL) Guwahati

The Regional Drugs Testing Laboratory Guwahati is the one of the five National Laboratory of the Govt of India for quality control of Drugs and Cosmetic and is established under the Indian Drugs & Cosmetics Act 1940 functioning under administrative control of the Drugs Controller General of India and sub ordinate office under Directorate General of Health Services, Ministry of Health & Family Welfare. The laboratory was set up in the year 2002 for entire North Eastern State including Sikkim and is housed in its own building at Guwahati.

1. Statutory Function

a. Analytical quality control of drugs and cosmetic manufactured within the country on behalf of the Central and State Drugs Controller Administration.

b. To assists the Central Drugs Standard Control Organization in the testing of Drugs and cosmetic.

Central Drug Laboratory, CRI Kasauli

Central drug laboratory at CRI Kasauli is a Central laboratory engaged in the testing of vaccines. It is a notified laboratory under the Drugs and cosmetics Act, 1940 to function as Central drugs laboratory for testing of the following drugs or classes of drugs;

i) Sera

ii) Solution of serum proteins intended for injection

iii) Vaccines

iv) Toxins

v) Antigens

vi) Anti-toxins

vii) Sterilized surgical ligature and sterilized surgical suture

viii) Bacteriophages, including Oral Polio vaccine.

Function

The main functions of the CDSCO include control of the quality of drugs imported into the country, coordination of the activities of the States/U.Ts Drug Control Authorities, approval of new drugs proposed to be imported or manufactured in the country, laying down standards and regulatory measures and acting as the Central License Approving Authority (CLAA) in respect of whole human blood and its products, Large Volume Parenterals (IV Fluids), Sera and Vaccines,r-DNA products, Quality of cosmetics manufactured and marketed in the country are also regulated under the Drug & Cosmetic Act. The I.P. Committee under the CDSCO brings out the Indian Pharmacopoeia which lays down the National Standards for drugs and formulations.

Functions undertaken by Central Government

Statutory Functions

➤ Laying down standards of drugs, cosmetics, diagnostics and devices.

➤ Laying down regulatory measures, amendments to Acts and Rules.

➤ To regulate market authorization of new drugs.

➤ Work relating to the Drugs Technical Advisory Board (DTAB) and Drugs Consultative Committee (DCC).

➤ Testing of drugs by Central Drugs Labs.

➤ Publication of Indian Pharmacopoeia.

Other Functions

➤ Coordinating the activities of the State Drugs Control Organizations to achieve uniform administration of the Act; and policy guidance.

➤ Guidance on technical matters.

➤ Participation in the WHO GMP certification scheme.

➤ Monitoring adverse drug reactions (ADR).

➤ Conducting training programmes for regulatory officials & Govt. Analysts.

➤ Distribution of quotas of narcotic drugs for use in medicinal formulations.

➤ Screening of drug formulations available in Indian market.

➤ Evaluation/Screening of applications for granting No Objection Certificates for export of unapproved/banned drugs.

Functions undertaken by State Governments

Statutory Functions

➤ Licensing of drug manufacturing and sales establishments.

> ➤ Licensing of drug testing laboratories.

> ➤ Approval of drug formulations for manufacture.

> ➤ Monitoring of quality of Drugs & Cosmetics, manufactured by respective state units and those marketed in the state.

> ➤ Investigation and prosecution in respect of contravention of legal provisions.

> ➤ Administrative actions.

> ➤ Pre- and post- licensing inspection.

> ➤ Recall of sub-standard drugs.

5.3 US FDA

The Food and Drug Administration (FDA or USFDA) is an agency of the United States Department of Health and Human Services, one of the United States federal executive departments, responsible for protecting and promoting public health through the regulation and supervision of food safety, tobacco products, dietary supplements, prescription and over-the-counter pharmaceutical drugs (medications), vaccines, biopharmaceuticals, blood transfusions, medical devices, electromagnetic radiation emitting devices (ERED), veterinary products, and cosmetics.

The FDA is led by a Commissioner of Food and Drugs, appointed by the President with the advice and consent of the Senate. The Commissioner reports to the Secretary of Health and Human Services. The FDA has its headquarters at Silver Spring, Maryland and has 223 field offices and 13 laboratories located throughout the 50 states. In 2008 the FDA started opening offices in foreign countries, including China, India, Costa Rica, Chile, Belgium, and the United Kingdom.

Organization

The FDA comprises several offices and centers. There are

> ➤ Office of the Commissioner

> ➤ Center for Biologics Evaluation and Research

> ➤ Center for Devices and Radiological Health (CDRH)

- ✓ Office of the Center Director
- ✓ Office of Communication, Education, and Radiation Programs
- ✓ Office of Compliance
- ✓ Office of Device Evaluation
- ✓ Office of In Vitro Diagnostic Device Evaluation and Safety
- ✓ Office of Management Operations
- ✓ Office of Science and Engineering Laboratories
- ✓ Office of Surveillance and Biometrics

➤ **Center for Drug Evaluation and Research (CDER)**

- ✓ Office of the Center Director.
  - Advisory Committee Staff.
  - Controlled Substance Staff.
- ✓ Office of Compliance.
  - Division of Compliance Risk Management and Surveillance.
  - Division of Manufacturing and Product Quality.
  - Division of New Drugs and Labeling Compliance.
  - Division of Scientific Investigations.

➤ Office of Medical Policy.

- ✓ Division of Drug Marketing, Advertising and Communications.

➤ Office of New Drugs.

➤ Office of Nonprescription Products.

➤ Office of Oncology Drug Products.

- ✓ Radioactive Drug Research Committee (RDRC) Program.

- Office of Pharmaceutical Science.
  - ✓ Office of Biotechnology Products.
  - ✓ Office of Generic Drugs.
  - ✓ Office of New Drug Quality Assessment.
  - ✓ Office of Testing and Research.
  - ✓ Division of Applied Pharmacology Research.
  - ✓ Division of Pharmaceutical Analysis.
  - ✓ Division of Product Quality Research.
  - ✓ Informatics and Computational Safety Analysis Staff (ICSAS).
- Office of Surveillance and Epidemiology (formerly Office of Drug Safety).
- Office of Translational Sciences.
  - ✓ Office of Biostatistics.
  - ✓ Office of Clinical Pharmacology.
  - ✓ Pharmacometrics Staff.
- Division of Drug Information.
  - ✓ FDA Pharmacy Student Experiential Program.
- Botanical Review Team.
- Maternal Health Team.
  - ✓ Center for Food Safety and Applied Nutrition.
  - ✓ Center for Tobacco Products.
  - ✓ Center for Veterinary Medicine.
  - ✓ National Center for Toxicological Research.
  - ✓ Office of Regulatory Affairs.

In recent years the agency began undertaking a large-scale effort to consolidate its operations in the Washington Metropolitan Area from its main headquarters in Rockville and several fragmented office buildings in the vicinity to the former site of the Naval Ordnance Laboratory in the White Oak area of Silver Spring, Maryland. When the FDA arrived, the site was renamed from the White Oak Naval Surface Warfare Center to the Federal Research Center at White Oak. The first building, the Life Sciences Laboratory, was dedicated and opened with 104 employees on the campus in December 2003. The project is slated to be completed by 2013.

While most of the Centers are located around the Washington, D.C., area as part of the Headquarters divisions, two offices - the Office of Regulatory Affairs (ORA) and the Office of Criminal Investigations (OCI) - are primarily field offices with a workforce spread across the country.

The Office of Regulatory Affairs is considered the "eyes and ears" of the agency, conducting the vast majority of the FDA's work in the field. Consumer Safety Officers, more commonly called Investigators, are the individuals who inspect production and warehousing facilities, investigate complaints, illnesses, or outbreaks, and review documentation in the case of medical devices, drugs, biological products, and other items where it may be difficult to conduct a physical examination or take a physical sample of the product. The Office of Regulatory Affairs is divided into five regions, which are further divided into 13 districts. Districts are based roughly on the geographic divisions of the federal court system. Each district comprises a main district office, and a number of Resident Posts, which are FDA offices located away from the district office to serve a particular geographic area. ORA also includes the Agency's network of laboratories, which analyze any physical samples taken. Though samples are usually food-related, some laboratories are equipped to analyze drugs, cosmetics, and radiation-emitting devices.

The Office of Criminal Investigations was established in 1991 to investigate criminal cases. Unlike ORA Investigators, OCI Special Agents are armed, and are not focused on the technical aspects of the regulated industries. OCI agents pursue and develop cases where criminal actions have occurred, such as fraudulent claims, or knowingly and willfully shipping known adulterated goods in interstate commerce. In many cases, OCI will pursue cases where Title 18 violations have occurred (e.g. conspiracy, false statements, wire fraud, mail fraud), in addition to prohibited acts as defined in Chapter III of the FD&C Act. OCI Special Agents often come from other criminal investigations backgrounds, and work closely with the Federal Bureau of Investigation, Assistant Attorney General, and even Interpol. OCI will receive cases from a variety of sources, including ORA, local agencies, and the FBI, and will work with ORA investigators to help develop the technical and science-based aspects of a case. OCI is a smaller branch, comprising of about 200 agents nationwide.

The FDA frequently works in conjunction with other federal agencies including the Department of Agriculture, Drug Enforcement Administration, Customs and Border Protection, and Consumer Product Safety Commission. Often local and state government agencies also work in cooperation with the FDA to provide regulatory inspections and enforcement action.

New drugs

New drugs receive extensive scrutiny before FDA approval in a process called a New Drug Application or NDA. New drugs are available only by prescription by default. A change to Over the Counter (OTC) status is a separate process and the drug must be approved through an NDA first. A drug that is approved is said to be "safe and effective when used as directed."

Post market safety surveillance

After approval of an NDA, the sponsor must review and report to the FDA every patient adverse drug experience of which it learns. Unexpected serious and fatal adverse drug events must be reported within 15 days; other events on a quarterly basis. The FDA also receives directly adverse drug event reports through its MedWatch program. These reports are called '"spontaneous reports" because reporting by consumers and health professionals is voluntary. While this remains the primary tool of postmarket safety surveillance, FDA requirements for postmarketing risk management are increasing. As a condition of approval, a sponsor may be required to conduct additional clinical trials, called Phase IV trials. In some cases the FDA requires risk management plans for some drugs that may provide for other kinds of studies, restrictions, or safety surveillance activities.

Generic drugs

Generic drugs are chemical equivalents of name-brand drugs whose patents have expired. Generally they are less expensive than their name brand counterparts, are manufactured and marketed by other companies and, in the 1990s, accounted for about a third of all prescriptions written in the United States. For approval of a generic drug, the U.S. Food and Drug Administration (FDA) requires scientific evidence that the generic drug is interchangeable or therapeutically equivalent with the originally approved drug. This is called an "ANDA" (Abbreviated New Drug Application).

Over-the-counter drugs

Over-the-counter (OTC) drugs are drugs and combinations that do not require a doctor's prescription. Many OTC drug ingredients had been previously approved prescription drugs now deemed safe enough for use without a medical practitioner's supervision.

Post-marketing drug safety monitoring

The widely publicized recall of Vioxx, a non-steroidal anti-inflammatory drug now estimated to have contributed to fatal heart attacks in thousands of Americans, played a strong role in driving a new wave of safety reforms at both the FDA rulemaking and statutory levels. Vioxx was approved by the FDA in 1999, and was initially hoped to be safer than previous NSAIDs, due to its reduced risk of intestinal tract bleeding. However, a number of pre- and post-marketing studies suggested that Vioxx might increase the risk of myocardial infarction, and this was conclusively demonstrated by results from the APPROVE trial in 2004. Faced with numerous lawsuits, the manufacturer voluntarily withdrew it from the market. The example of Vioxx has been prominent in an ongoing debate over whether new drugs should be evaluated on the basis of their absolute safety, or their safety relative to existing treatments for a given condition. In the wake of the Vioxx recall, there were widespread calls by major newspapers, medical journals, consumer advocacy organizations, lawmakers, and FDA officials for reforms in the FDA's procedures for pre- and post- market drug safety regulation.

In 2006, a congressionally requested committee was appointed by the Institute of Medicine to review pharmaceutical safety regulation in the U.S. and to issue recommendations for improvements. The committee was composed of 16 experts, including leaders in clinical medicinemedical research, economics, biostatistics, law, public policy, public health, and the allied health professions, as well as current and former executives from the pharmaceutical, hospital, and health insurance industries. The authors found major deficiencies in the current FDA system for ensuring the safety of drugs on the American market. Overall, the authors called for an increase in the regulatory powers, funding, and independence of the FDA. Some of the committee's recommendations have been incorporated into drafts of the PDUFA IV bill which was signed into law in 2007.

5.4 AUSTRALIAN TGA

INTRODUCTION

The Act sets out the legal requirements for the import, export, manufacture and supply of medicines in Australia. It details the requirements for listing or registering all medicines on the Australian Register of Therapeutic Goods (ARTG), as well as many other aspects of the law including advertising, labelling, and product appearance. The Act is supported by the Regulations, and various Orders and Determinations which provide further details of matters covered in the Act. The Act is a Commonwealth Act that provides a substantially uniform national system of controls over therapeutic goods, facilitating trade between the States/Territories and benefiting both consumers and industry.

The Australian Register of Therapeutic Goods (ARTG) has been established under Section 17 of the

Therapeutic Goods Act 1989 for compiling information in relation to, and providing for, the evaluation of therapeutic goods for use in humans. Its role is to provide a comprehensive data base of information about all therapeutic goods supplied in Australia or exported from Australia. TGA has developed and maintains lists of Australian Approved terminology, to ensure accuracy and consistency in the information compiled in the ARTG. For medicines, the lists cover substances (active ingredients and excipients), containers, dosage forms, routes of administration and units of expression and proportion. These lists are reproduced in this publication. Australian Approved terminology has been developed by the Therapeutic Goods Administration as no single internationally agreed list or primary reference is available which covers comprehensively all substances or terms used, or likely to be used in therapeutic goods in Australia.

Role of the TGA

The TGA carries out a range of assessment and monitoring activities to ensure that all therapeutic goods available in Australia are of an acceptable standard. At the same time, the TGA aims to ensure that the Australian community has access, within a reasonable time, to therapeutic advances.

Overall control of medicines is exerted through five main processes:

- pre-market evaluation and approval of registered products intended for supply in Australia

- development, maintenance and monitoring of the systems for listing of medicines

- licensing of manufacturers in accordance with international standards of Good Manufacturing Practice;

- post-market monitoring, through sampling, adverse event reporting, surveillance activities, and response to public inquiries; and

- the assessment of medicines for export.

Australian Register of Therapeutic Goods (ARTG)

The Australian Register of Therapeutic Goods (ARTG) has been established under Section 17 of the *Therapeutic Goods Act 1989* for compiling information in relation to, and providing for, theevaluation of therapeutic goods for use in humans. Its role is to provide a comprehensive data base of information about all therapeutic goods supplied in Australia or exported from Australia.

TGA has developed and maintains lists of Australian Approved terminology, to ensure accuracy and consistency in the information compiled in the ARTG. For medicines, the lists cover substances (active ingredients and excipients), containers, dosage forms, routes of administration and units of expression and proportion. These lists are reproduced in this publication.

Australian Approved terminology has been developed by the Therapeutic Goods Administration as no single internationally agreed list or primary reference is available which covers comprehensively all substances or terms used, or likely to be used in therapeutic goods in Australia.

Australian Approved terminology should be used:

1. When submitting applications for registration or listing of medicines

2. In drug formulation records included in the Australian Register of Therapeutic Goods (ARTG)

3. On labels, in accordance with the requirements of Therapeutic Goods Order (TGO) 48 – *General Requirements for Labels for Drug Products* (as amended)

4. In product information, consumer medicine information and other promotional literature where use of approved terminology is required. Consistency in naming assists the retrieval of information from the ARTG and the ability of health professionals and the public to compare similar goods. Although disinfectants and sterilants are classified as therapeutic devices, TGO 54 and 54A – *Standard for Composition, Packaging, Labelling and Performance of Disinfectants and Sterilants* require the use of terminology as published in the *TGA Approved Terminology for Medicines*. Thus a section devoted to substances names

eligible for use in devices has been included within the Chemical Substances Section.

Regulation of therapeutic goods in Australia

The Australian community expects that medicines and medical devices in the marketplace are safe and of high quality, and of a standard at least equal to that of comparable countries. The objective of the Therapeutic Goods Act 1989, which came into effect on 15 February 1991, is to provide a national framework for the regulation of therapeutic goods in Australia to ensure the quality, safety and efficacy of medicines and ensure the quality, safety and performance of medical devices.

The regulatory framework is based on a risk management approach designed to ensure public health and safety, while at the same time freeing industry from any unnecessary regulatory burden.

Essentially therapeutic goods must be entered on the <u>Australian Register of Therapeutic Goods (ARTG)</u> before they can be supplied in Australia. The ARTG is a computer database of information about therapeutic goods for human use approved for supply in, or exported from, Australia.

The Therapeutic Goods Act 1989, Regulations and Orders set out the requirements for inclusion of therapeutic goods in the ARTG, including advertising, labelling, product appearance and appeal guidelines. Some provisions such as the scheduling of substances and the safe storage of therapeutic goods, are covered by the relevant State or Territory legislation.

The Therapeutic Goods Administration (TGA) is a unit of the Australian Government Department of Health and Ageing and is responsible for administering the provisions of the legislation.

The TGA carries out a range of assessment and monitoring activities to ensure therapeutic goods available in Australia are of an acceptable standard. At the same time the TGA aims to ensure that the Australian community has access, within a reasonable time, to therapeutic advances.

What is a therapeutic good?

A 'therapeutic good' is broadly defined as a good which is represented in any way to be, or is likely to be taken to be, for therapeutic use (unless specifically excluded or included under Section 7 of the Therapeutic Goods Act 1989).

Therapeutic use means use in or in connection with:

- preventing, diagnosing, curing or alleviating a disease, ailment, defect or injury;
- influencing inhibiting or modifying a physiological process;
- testing the susceptibility of persons to a disease or ailment;
- influencing, controlling or preventing conception;
- testing for pregnancy; or
- replacement or modification of parts of the anatomy.

Overall control of the supply of therapeutic goods is exercised through three main processes

- Auditing and assessment of the quality of their manufacture.
- Pre-market assessment of the goods
- Post market monitoring of compliance with standards once the goods are supplied on the market.

Regulation of advertising of therapeutic goods in Australia.

Advertisements for therapeutic goods are subject to the requirements of the Therapeutic Goods Act 1989 ("the Act") and Regulations, the Trade Practices Act 1974 and other relevant laws. Additionally, advertisements for therapeutic goods directed to consumers must comply with the Therapeutic Goods Advertising Code (TGAC)

Advertisement, in relation to therapeutic goods, includes any statement, pictorial representation or design, however made, that is intended, whether directly or indirectly, to promote the use of supply of the goods (Therapeutic Goods Act 1989).

Section 22(5) of the Act specifies that advertising of a therapeutic good can only refer to the indications which are included in the Australian Register of Therapeutic Goods for that specific good.

Prescription only medicines

- Advertising direct to consumers is not permitted (prohibited by the Act).

- Advertising to healthcare professionals is permitted and is regulated by a self-regulatory scheme operated by Medicines Australia.

- Prior approval of advertisements is not applicable.

- Complaints about advertisements for prescription medicines directed to healthcare professionals are handled by Medicines Australia.

- TGA's letter of marketing approval requires the promotion of all prescription products (whether member or non-member) to comply with the requirements of the Medicines Australia Code of Conduct.

- If a complaint is made about the advertising activities of a non-member, the complaint is forwarded to the non-member with an invitation to have the complaint adjudicated by the Medicines Australia Code of Conduct Committee. If the non-member declines the invitation for adjudication, the Medicines Australia may forward the complaint to the Therapeutic Goods Administration (TGA) or the Australian Competition and Consumer Commission.

- Where it has been determined that a breach of the Code has occurred, the Committee may impose a range of fines, depending on the nature of the breach. The Committee may also recommend to the Medicines Australia Board that a member be suspended or expelled.

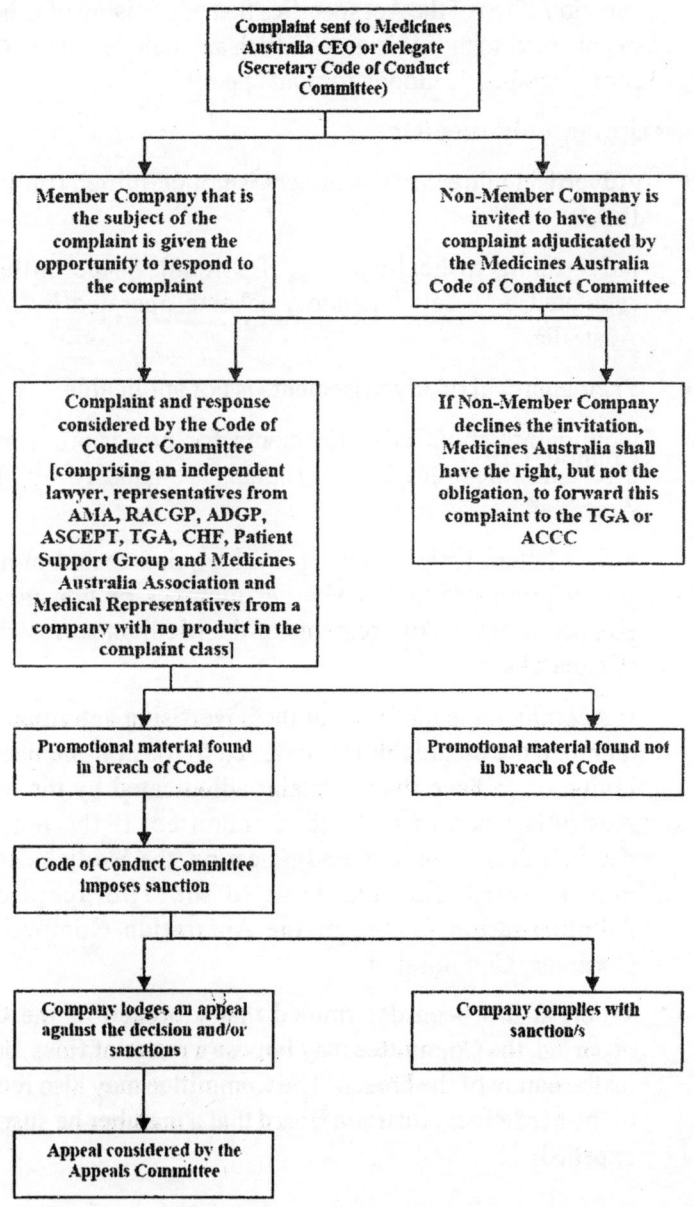

Fig.1: Medicines Australia Promotion of Prescription Medicines to Healthcare Professionals Complaints Handling Process.

Non-prescription medicines

- Non-prescription medicines are over-the-counter (OTC) medicines and non-prescription complementary medicines.

- Generally, advertisements for non-prescription medicines may be directed both to consumers and to healthcare professionals. However, the Regulations also prohibit the advertising to consumers of certain goods included in Schedule 3 of the Standard for the Uniform Scheduling of Drugs and Poisons. Advertisements for non-prescription medicines are regulated by both co-regulatory and self-regulatory arrangements operated by the TGA, the Therapeutic Goods Advertising Code Council, the Australian Self-Medication Industry (ASMI) and the Complementary Healthcare Council (CHC).

- Certain types of advertisements directed to consumers require prior approval by a Delegate of the Secretary of the Department of Health and Ageing.

Organization of TGA

The Therapeutic Goods Administration (TGA) is a division of the Australian Government Department of Health and Ageing. The TGA regulatory offices are grouped into three core groups – Market Authorisation Group, Monitoring and Compliance Group and Regulatory Support Group.

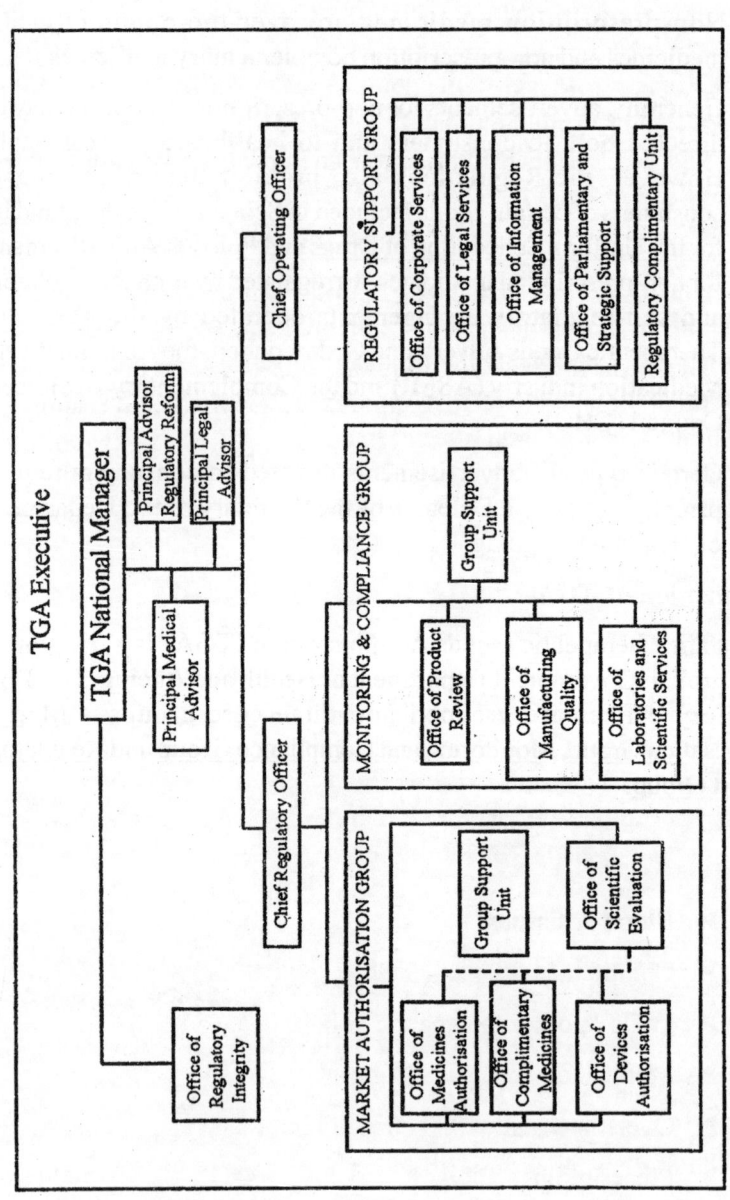

Fig.2. Therapeutic Goods Administaration

TGA Executive

The TGA Executive has overall responsibility for the management of the TGA's regulatory functions and activities.

Market Authorisation Group

The Marketing Authorisation Group is responsible for the evaluation and authorisation of therapeutic goods to ensure they meet appropriate standards of quality, safety and efficacy or performance, consistent with their risk.

Monitoring and Compliance Group

The Monitoring and Compliance Group is responsible for monitoring of therapeutic goods on the Australian market to ensure that they comply with required standards of quality, safety, efficacy and performance.

Regulatory Support Group

The Regulatory Support Group provides the business systems and support services that enable the TGA to undertake its regulatory responsibilities.

Office of Regulatory Integrity

The Office of Regulatory Integrity functions as an internal auditor of regulatory activity and advises the TGA Executive on the appropriate operation of regulatory frameworks across the TGA.

Regulation Of TGA

➢ Blood & tissues

➢ Complementary medicines

➢ IVDs & other therapeutic goods

➢ Medical devices

➢ Over-the-counter (OTC) medicines

➢ Prescription medicines

5.5 CANADIAN HPFBI

Introduction

Health Products and Food Branch Inspectorate (HPFBI) of Health Canada to protect the health and safety of Canadians. Although manufacturers and importers are required to report medical device problems, the HPFBI encourages anyone purchasing, using or maintaining these products to report problems.

Reporting of problems can result in the prevention of similar problems and in some cases has led to product modifications, redesign, recalls, or improvements in directions for use. In addition, this information could lead to the issuance of a warning or Medical Device Alert. Failure to notify the manufacturer and the HPFBI could place patients at risk at other facilities that are not aware of the problem. In general, medical device problem reporting contributes to an increased level of device safety, effectiveness and quality.

Any concerns that relate to the safety, effectiveness or quality of a medical device that have been detected during use or identified during device examination and testing prior to use should be reported. The problems include deficiencies in the design of the device, defects arising from the manufacturing and inadequacy or errors in labeling such as directions for use.

After the details of the incident have been verified with the user, the information will be entered into the national incident database. Depending on the problem report details, a Health Canada inspector may visit the user to examine the device and to take samples, if necessary. The Health Canada Regional Office that is responsible for the manufacturer or importer of the medical device in question will be notified. They will follow-up with the manufacturer or importer as needed depending on the level of risk associated with the continued use of the device.

The HPFBI acts as a central clearing house for problem report data, and can link isolated reports to identify problems that would otherwise go unnoticed or dismissed as an isolated incident. Once assessed by the manufacturer in consultation with the HPFBI, all affected facilities and professionals can be promptly informed of the situation and required actions.

In addition, the HPFBI

➤ Provides inspectors across Canada to assist users in investigating medical device problems;

➤ Monitors the manufacturer's investigation and steps taken to correct the problem to ensure they are adequate to establish the safety and effectiveness of the device

➤ Provides assistance from scientific, medical and engineering staff to identify the cause of problems and possible solutions, which may include testing of devices;

➤ Provides access to Health Canada's expertise in risk identification and management;

➤ Assists in determining device compliance with other regulatory requirements such as medical device licensing;

➤ Issues Medical Devices Alerts to advise health care facilities and other users of problems with a medical device, when intervention is required; and

➤ In cases where a manufacturer is not prepared to take sufficient steps to correct a problem, the HPFBI will take action to ensure that the safety of users and patients is not jeopardized.

Call the Inspectorate Hotline number to reach a Medical Device Inspector in your Region. After reviewing the details of the incident, the inspector may ask you to complete the HPFBI's problem reporting form and fax it to their office. This form along with a guidance document on Voluntary and Mandatory Problem Reporting are available on the website.

5.6 INTRODUCTION TO NDA & ANDA

New Drug Application(NDA)

The **New Drug Application** (NDA) is the vehicle in the United States through which drug sponsors formally propose that the FDA approve a new pharmaceutical for sale and marketing. The goals of the

NDA are to provide enough information to permit FDA reviewers to establish the following:

- Is the drug safe and effective in its proposed use(s) when used as directed, and do the benefits of the drug outweigh the risks.

- Is the drug's proposed labeling (package insert) appropriate, and what should it contain.

- Are the methods used in manufacturing (Good Manufacturing Practice, GMP) the drug and the controls used to maintain the drug's quality adequate to preserve the drug's identity, strength, quality, and purity.

For decades, the regulation and control of new drugs in the United States has been based on the New Drug Application (NDA). Since 1938, every new drug has been the subject of an approved NDA before U.S. commercialization. The NDA application is the vehicle through which drug sponsors formally propose that the FDA approve a new pharmaceutical for sale and marketing in the U.S. The data gathered during the animal studies and human clinical trials of an Investigational New Drug (IND) become part of the NDA.

The goals of the NDA are to provide enough information to permit FDA reviewer to reach the following key decisions:

- Whether the drug is safe and effective in its proposed use(s), and whether the benefits of the drug outweigh the risks.

- Whether the drug's proposed labeling (package insert) is appropriate, and what it should contain.

- Whether the methods used in manufacturing the drug and the controls used to maintain the drug's quality are adequate to preserve the drug's identity, strength, quality, and purity.

The documentation required in an NDA is supposed to tell the drug's whole story, including what happened during the clinical tests, what the ingredients of the drug are, the results of the animal studies, how the drug behaves in the body, and how it is manufactured, processed and packaged.

New Drug Application (NDA) Process

For decades, the regulation and control of new drugs in the United States has been based on the New Drug Application (NDA). Since 1938, every new drug or therapy has been the subject of an approved NDA before US commercialization. The NDA application is the vehicle through which drug sponsors, such as biotech and pharmaceutical companies, formally propose that the FDA approve a new pharmaceutical for sale and marketing in the US. The data gathered during the animal studies and human clinical trials of an Investigational New Drug (IND) become part of the NDA.

The goals of the NDA are to provide enough information to permit FDA reviewers to reach the following key decisions:

➤ Whether the drug is safe and effective in its propose use(s), and whether the benefits of the drug outweigh the risks.

➤ Whether the drug's proposed labeling (package insert) is appropriate, and what it should contain.

➤ Whether the methods used in manufacturing the drug and the controls used to maintain the drug's quality are adequate to preserve the drug's identity, strength, quality, and purity.

The documentation required in an NDA is supposed to tell the drug's whole story, including what happened during the clinical tests, what the ingredients of the drug are, the results of the animal studies, how the drug behaves in the body, and how it is manufactured, processed and packaged. **FDA Drug Review and Approval Time** FDA is often asked about the pace of drug approvals and how FDA review time for applications affects it. Since the Prescription Drug User Fee Act (PDUFA) was passed in 1992, FDA has met and often exceeded the vast majority of review-time goals established under the Act. New drug approval times also have been dramatically reduced (from a median of 22 months in 1992 to a median of less than 12 months in 1999), although a slight increase was seen for the year 2000.

Definitions FDA Review Time: The time it takes FDA to review a new drug application. Review time goals are established under PDUFA.

Approval Time: Approval time is the time from first NDA submission to NDA approval. It includes the sum of: FDA review time for the first submission of an NDA to the Agency, plus any subsequent time during which a pharmaceutical sponsor addresses deficiencies in the NDA and resubmits the application, plus subsequent FDA review time.

New Molecular Entity (NME): A medication containing an active substance that has never before been approved for marketing in any form in the United States.

Priority New Drug Application (NDA): An application for a product determined to provide a significant therapeutic or public health advance. Priority NDAs have a 6-month FDA review performance goal.

Standard New Drug Application (NDA): A NDA for a product that is not designated as a Priority NDA. The performance goal for FDA review for a standard NDA is 10-12 months.

FDA Approvable: The FDA has essentially approved the product but remaining questions will need to answered by the sponsor before an actual approval is received. Typically, the sponsor replies within three months with another three months for final review by the FDA. Therefore, the product would be approved for availability and marketing in the US six (6) months after receiving an FDA approvable. FDA Approval: The sponsor has received final product approval by the FDA to sell and market a product in the US with no exceptions and/or questions.

The number of Priority NMEs, those with a 6-month review goal, reviewed in a given year impacts the median approval time for drugs. In 1999, 19 of 35 (54%) NMEs had priority designation. For 2000, only 9 of 27 (33%) of the NMEs had priority designation. By definition, a drug's time to approval includes time that the NDA is under review by FDA, as well as any time it takes the pharmaceutical sponsor to address deficiencies identified by the FDA. Deficiencies can range from requiring new data analyses, to product labeling revisions, to the need for conducting additional clinical studies. Some applications go through more than one cycle of NDA submission followed by an FDA action other than approval. The percentage of NMEs that are approved within 12 months of submission has remained relatively constant in recent years at around 40%. However, products with longer regulatory NDA histories with multiple review cycles can significantly affect aggregate time to approval for drugs in a given year.

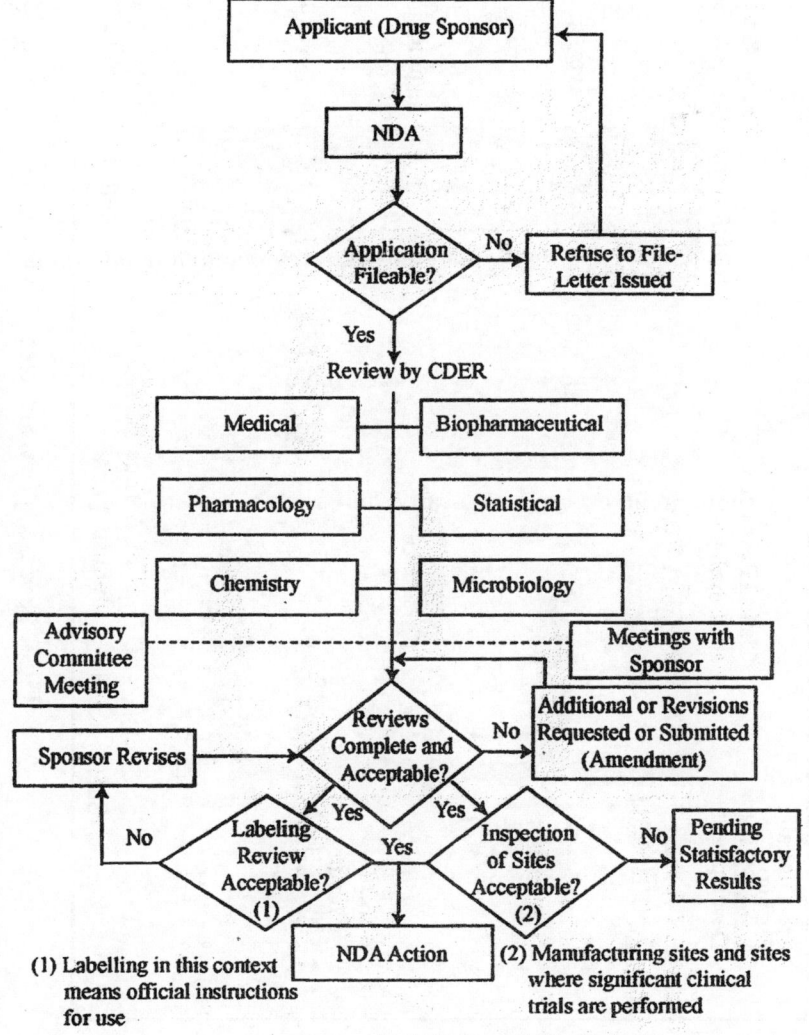

Fig.3: NDA Review Process

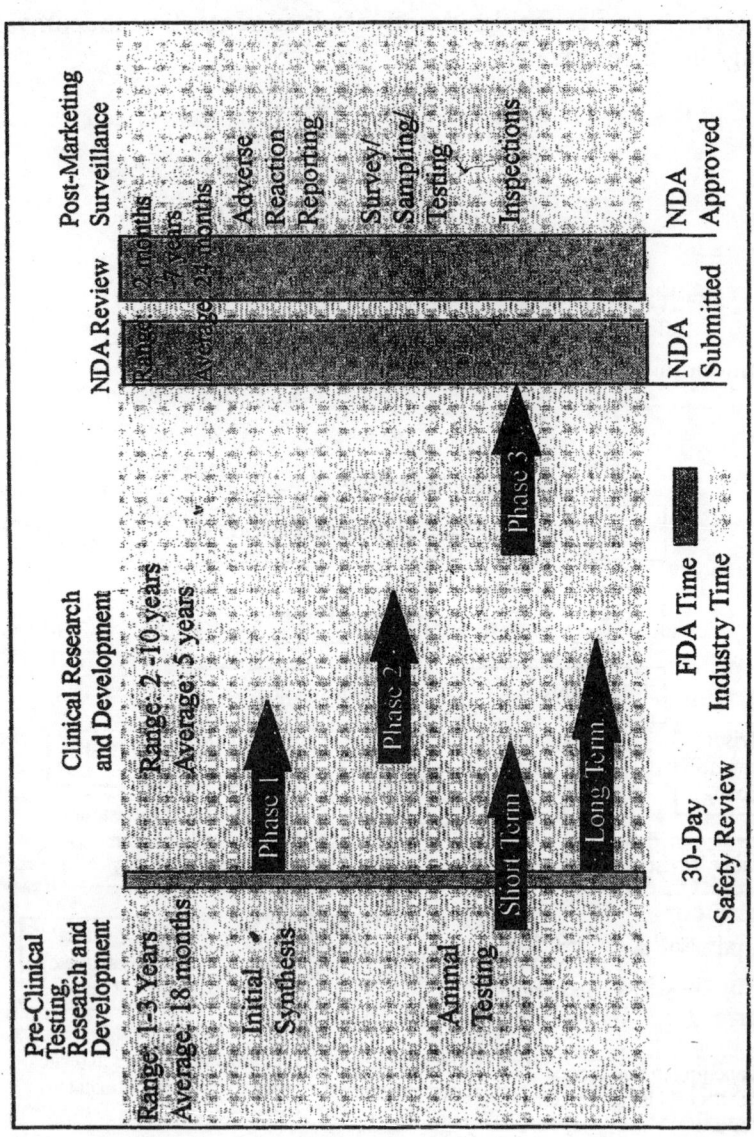

Fig.4. New Drug Development Timeline

5.7 ABBREVIATED NEW DRUG APPLICATION (ANDA) GENERICS

An **Abbreviated New Drug Application** (ANDA) is an application for a U.S. generic drug approval for an existing licensed medication or approved drug. An Abbreviated New Drug Application (ANDA) contains data which when submitted to FDA's Center for Drug Evaluation and Research, Office of Generic Drugs, provides for the review and ultimate approval of a generic drug product. Once approved, an applicant may manufacture and market the generic drug product to provide a safe, effective, low cost alternative to the American public.

A generic drug product is one that is comparable to an innovator drug product in dosage form, strength, route of administration, quality, performance characteristics and intended use. All approved products, both innovator and generic, are listed in FDA's *Approved Drug Products with Therapeutic Equivalence Evaluations* (*Orange Book*).

Generic drug applications are termed "abbreviated" because they are generally not required to include preclinical (animal) and clinical (human) data to establish safety and effectiveness. Instead, generic applicants must scientifically demonstrate that their product is bioequivalent (i.e., performs in the same manner as the innovator drug). One way scientists demonstrate bioequivalence is to measure the time it takes the generic drug to reach the bloodstream in 24 to 36 healthy, volunteers. This gives them the rate of absorption, or bioavailability, of the generic drug, which they can then compare to that of the innovator drug. The generic version must deliver the same amount of active ingredients into a patient's bloodstream in the same amount of time as the innovator drug. Using bioequivalence as the basis for approving generic copies of drug products was established by the "Drug Price Competition and Patent Term Restoration Act of 1984," also known as the Waxman-Hatch Act. This Act expedites the availability of less costly generic drugs by permitting FDA to approve applications to market generic versions of brand-name drugs without conducting costly and duplicative clinical trials. At the same time, the brand-name companies can apply for up to five additional years longer patent protection for the new medicines they developed to make up for time lost while their products were going through FDA's approval process. Brand-name drugs are subject to the same bioequivalence tests as generics upon reformulation.

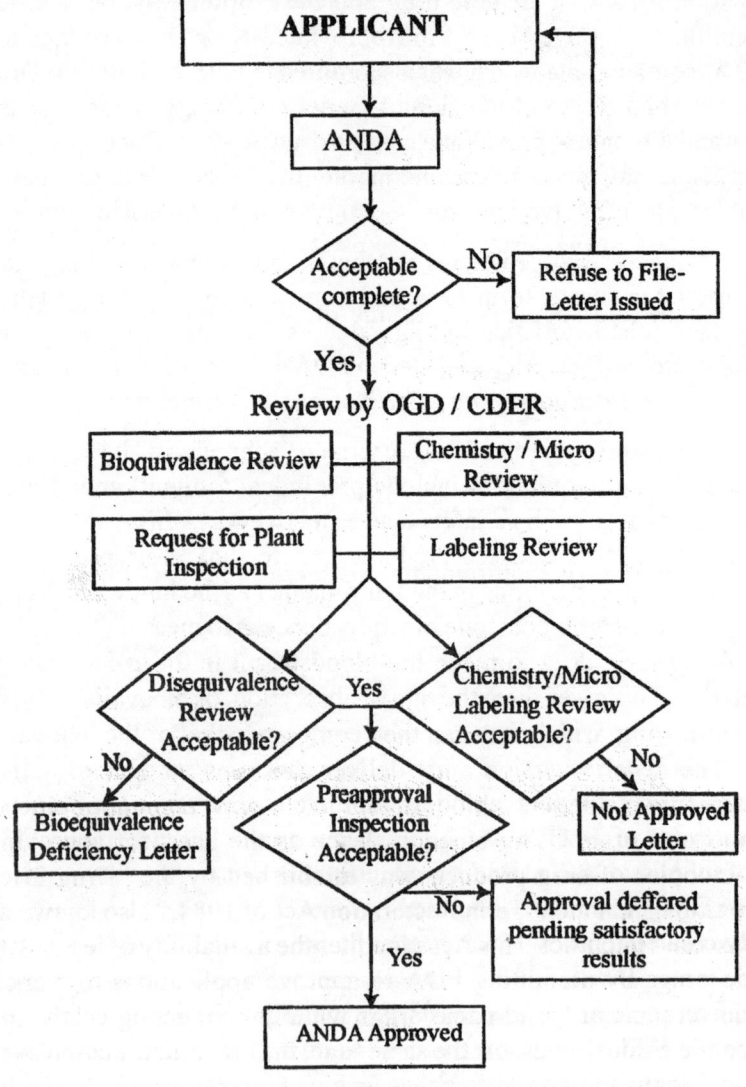

Fig.5. Generic Drug (ANDA) Review Process

5.8 GUIDELINE FOR DRUG MASTER FILES

I. INTRODUCTION

A Drug Master File (DMF) is a submission to the Food and Drug Administration (FDA) that may be used to provide confidential detailed information about facilities, processes, or articles used in the manufacturing, processing, packaging, and storing of one or more human drugs. The submission of a DMF is not required by law or FDA regulation. A DMF is submitted solely at the discretion of the holder. The information contained in the DMF may be used to support an Investigational New Drug Application (IND), a New Drug Application (NDA), an Abbreviated New Drug Application (ANDA), another DMF, an Export Application, or amendments and supplements to any of these. A DMF is NOT a substitute for an IND, NDA, ANDA, or Export Application. It is not approved or disapproved. Technical contents of a DMF are reviewed only in connection with the review of an IND, NDA, ANDA, or an Export Application.

This guideline does not impose mandatory requirements (21 CFR 10.90(b)). It does, however, offer guidance on acceptable approaches to meeting regulatory requirements. Different approaches may be followed, but the applicant is encouraged to discuss significant variations in advance with FDA reviewers to preclude spending time and effort in preparing a submission that FDA may later determine to be unacceptable.

Drug Master Files are provided for in 21 CFR 314.420. This guideline is intended to provide DMF holders with procedures acceptable to the agency for preparing and submitting a DMF. The guideline discusses types of DMF's, the information needed in each type, the format of submissions to a DMF, the administrative procedures governing review of DMF's, and the obligations of the DMF holder. DMF's are generally created to allow a party other than the holder of the DMF to reference material without disclosing to that party the contents of the file. When an applicant references its own material, the applicant should reference the information contained in its own IND, NDA, or ANDA directly rather than establishing a new DMF.

II. DEFINITIONS

For the purposes of this guideline, the following definitions apply:

II.1. *Agency* means the Food and Drug Administration.

II.2 *Agent or representative* means any person who is appointed by a DMF holder to serve as the contact for the holder.

II.3. *Applicant* means any person who submits an application or abbreviated application or an amendment or supplement to them to obtain FDA approval of a new drug or an antibiotic drug and any other person who owns an approved application (21 CFR 314.3 (b)).

II.4. *Drug product* means a finished dosage form, for example, tablet, capsule, or solution, that contains a drug substance, generally, but not necessarily, in association with one or more other ingredients (21 CFR 314.3 (b)).

II.5. *Drug substance* means an active ingredient that is intended to furnish pharmacological   activity or other direct effect in the diagnosis, cure, mitigation, treatment, or prevention of disease or to affect the structure or any function of the human body, but does not include intermediates used in the synthesis of such ingredient (21 CFR 314.3 (b)).

II.6. *Export application* means an application submitted under section 802 of the Federal Food, Drug, and Cosmetic Act to export a drug that is not approved for marketing in the United States.

II.7. *Holder* means a person who owns a DMF.

II.8. *Letter of authorization* means a written statement by the holder or designated agent or representative permitting FDA to refer to information in the DMF in support of another person's submission.

II.9. *Person* includes individual, partnership, corporation, and association. (Section 201(e) of the Federal Food, Drug, and Cosmetic Act.)

II.10. *Sponsor* means a person who takes responsibility for and initiates a clinical investigation. The sponsor may be an individual or pharmaceutical company, governmental agency, academic institution, private organization, or other organization (21 CFR 312.3 (b)).

III. TYPES OF DRUG MASTER FILES

There are five types of DMF's

Type I Manufacturing Site, Facilities, Operating Procedures, and Personnel

Type II Drug Substance, Drug Substance Intermediate, and Material Used in Their Preparation, or Drug Product

Type III Packaging Material

Type IV Excipient, Colorant, Flavor, Essence, or Material Used in Their Preparation

Type V FDA Accepted Reference Information

Each DMF should contain only one type of information and all supporting data. See Section IV.C of the guideline for more detailed descriptions of the kind of information desired in each type. Supporting information and data in a DMF can be cross referenced to any other DMF (see Part V).

IV. SUBMISSIONS TO DRUG MASTER FILES

Each DMF submission should contain a transmittal letter, administrative information about the submission, and the specific information to be included in the DMF as described in this section.

The DMF must be in the English language. Whenever a submission contains information in another language, an accurate certified English translation must also be included.

Each page of each copy of the DMF should be dated and consecutively numbered. An updated table of contents should be included with each submission.

IV. A. Transmittal Letters

The following should be included:

IV. A.1. Original Submissions

a. Identification of submission: Original, the type of DMF as classified in Section III, and its subject.

b. Identification of the applications, if known, that the DMF is intended to support, including the name and address of each sponsor, applicant, or holder, and all relevant document numbers.

c. Signature of the holder or the authorized representative.

d. Typewritten name and title of the signer.

IV. A. 2. Amendments

a. Identification of submission: Amendment, the DMF number, type of DMF, and the subject of the amendment.

b. A description of the purpose of submission, e.g., update, revised formula, or revised process.

c. Signature of the holder or the authorized representative.

d. Typewritten name and title of the signer.

IV. B. Administrative Information

Administrative information should include the following:

IV. B.1. Original Submissions

a. Names and addresses of the following:

(1) DMF holder.

(2) Corporate headquarters.

(3) Manufacturing/processing facility.

(4) Contact for FDA correspondence.

(5) Agent(s), if any.

b. The specific responsibilities of each person listed in any of the categories in Section a.

c. Statement of commitment.

A signed statement by the holder certifying that the DMF is current and that the DMF holder will comply with the statements made in it.

IV. B2. Amendments

a. Name of DMF holder.

b. DMF number.

c. Name and address for correspondence.

d. Affected section and/or page numbers of the DMF.

e. The name and address of each person whose IND, NDA, ANDA, DMF, or Export Application relies on the subject of the amendment for support.

f. The number of each IND, NDA, ANDA, DMF, and Export Application that relies on the subject of the amendment for support, if known.

g. Particular items within the IND, NDA, ANDA, DMF, and Export Application that are affected, if known.

IV. C. Drug Master File Contents

IV. C.1. Types of Drug Master Files

IV. C.1.a. *Type I*: Manufacturing Site, Facilities, Operating Procedures, and Personnel

A Type I DMF is recommended for a person outside of the United States to assist FDA in conducting on site inspections of their manufacturing facilities. The DMF should describe the manufacturing site, equipment capabilities, and operational layout.

A Type I DMF is normally not needed to describe domestic facilities, except in special cases, such as when a person is not registered and not routinely inspected.

The description of the site should include acreage, actual site address, and a map showing its location with respect to the nearest city. An aerial photograph and a diagram of the site may be helpful.

A diagram of major production and processing areas is helpful for understanding the operational layout. Major equipment should be described in terms of capabilities, application, and location. Make and model would not normally be needed unless the equipment is new or unique.

A diagram of major corporate organizational elements, with key manufacturing, quality control, and quality assurance positions highlighted, at both the manufacturing site and corporate headquarters, is also helpful.

IV. C.1.b.*Type II*: Drug Substance, Drug Substance Intermediate, and Material Used in Their Preparation, or Drug Product

A Type II DMF should, in general, be limited to a single drug intermediate, drug substance, drug product, or type of material used in their preparation.

IV. C.1.b.(1) Drug Substance Intermediates, Drug Substances, and Material Used in Their Preparation

Summarize all significant steps in the manufacturing and controls of the drug intermediate or substance. Detailed guidance on what should be included in a Type II DMF for drug substances and intermediates may be found in the following guidelines:

Guideline for Submitting Supporting Documentation in Drug Applications for the Manufacture of Drug Substances.

Guideline for the Format and Content of the Chemistry, Manufacturing, and Controls Section of an Application.

IV. C.1.b.(2) Drug Product

Manufacturing procedures and controls for finished dosage forms should ordinarily be submitted in an IND, NDA, ANDA, or Export Application. If this information cannot be submitted in an IND, NDA, ANDA, or Export Application, it should be submitted in a DMF. When a

Type II DMF is submitted for a drug product, the applicant/sponsor should follow the guidance provided in the following guidelines:

Guideline for the Format and Content of the Chemistry, Manufacturing, and Controls Section of an Application.

Guideline for Submitting Documentation for the Manufacture of and Controls for Drug Products

Guideline for Submitting Samples and Analytical Data for Methods Validation

IV. C.1.c.*Type III*: **Packaging Material**

Each packaging material should be identified by the intended use, components, composition, and controls for its release. The names of the suppliers or fabricators of the components used in preparing the packaging material and the acceptance specifications should also be given. Data supporting the acceptability of the packaging material for its intended use should also be submitted as outlined in the *"Guideline for Submitting Documentation for Packaging for Human Drugs and Biologics."*

Toxicological data on these materials would be included under this type of DMF, if not otherwise available by cross reference to another document.

IV. C.1.d.*Type IV* **Excipient, Colorant, Flavor, Essence, or Material Used in Their Preparation**

Each additive should be identified and characterized by its method of manufacture, release specifications, and testing methods.

Toxicological data on these materials would be included under this type of DMF, if not otherwise available by cross reference to another document.

Usually, the official compendia and FDA regulations for color additives (21 CFR Parts 70 through 82), direct food additives (21 CFR Parts 170 through 173), indirect food additives (21 CFR Parts 174 through 178), and food substances (21 CFR Parts 181 through 186) may be used as sources for release tests, specifications, and safety. Guidelines suggested for a Type II DMF may be helpful for preparing a Type IV DMF. The DMF should include any other supporting information and data that are not available by cross reference to another document.

IV. C.1.e.*Type V*: FDA Accepted Reference Information

FDA discourages the use of Type V DMF's for miscellaneous information, duplicate information, or information that should be included in one of the other types of DMF's. If any holder wishes to submit information and supporting data in a DMF that is not covered by Types I through IV, a holder must first submit a letter of intent to the Drug Master File Staff (for address, see D.5.a. of this section). FDA will then contact the holder to discuss the proposed submission.

IV. C.2. General Information and Suggestions

IV. C.2.a. Environmental Assessment

Type II, Type III, and Type IV DMF's should contain a commitment by the firm that its facilities will be operated in compliance with applicable environmental laws. If a completed environmental assessment is needed, see 21 CFR Part 25.

IV. C.2.b. Stability

Stability study design, data, interpretation, and other information should be submitted, when applicable, as outlined in the "*Guideline for Submitting Documentation for the Stability of Human Drugs and Biologics.*"

IV. D. Format, Assembly, and Delivery

IV. D.1.

An original and duplicate are to be submitted for all DMF submissions.

Drug Master File holders and their agents/representatives should retain a complete reference copy that is identical to, and maintained in the same chronological order as, their submissions to FDA.

IV. D.2.

The original and duplicate copies must be collated, fully assembled, and individually jacketed.

Each volume of a DMF should, in general, be no more than 2 inches thick. For multivolume submissions, number each volume. For example, for a 3 volume submission, the volumes would be numbered 1 of 3, 2 of 3, and 3 of 3.

IV. D.3.

U.S. standard paper size (8-1/2 by 11 inches) is preferred.

Paper length should not be less than 10 inches nor more than 12 inches. However, it may occasionally be necessary to use individual pages larger than standard paper size to present a floor plan, synthesis diagram, batch formula, or manufacturing instructions. Those pages should be folded and mounted to allow the page to be opened for review without disassembling the jacket and refolded without damage when the volume is shelved.

IV.D.4.

The agency's system for filing DMF's provides for assembly on the left side of the page. The left margin should be at least three fourths of an inch to assure that text is not obscured in the fastened area. The right margin should be at least one half of an inch. The submitter should punch holes 8 1/2 inches apart in each page.

V. AUTHORIZATION TO REFER TO A DRUG MASTER FILE

V. A. Letter of Authorization to FDA

Before FDA can review DMF information in support of an application, the DMF holder must submit in duplicate to the DMF a letter of authorization permitting FDA to reference the DMF. If the holder cross references its own DMF, the holder should supply in a letter of authorization the information designated by items 3, 5, 6, 7, and 8 of this section. The holder does not need to send a transmittal letter with its letter of authorization.

The letter of authorization should include the following:

1. The date.

2. Name of DMF holder.

3. DMF number.

4. Name of person(s) authorized to incorporate information in the DMF by reference.

5. Specific product(s) covered by the DMF.

6. Submission date(s) of 5, above.

7. Section numbers and/or page numbers to be referenced.

8. Statement of commitment that the DMF is current and that the DMF holder will comply with the statements made in it.

9. Signature of authorizing official.

10. Typed name and title of official authorizing reference to the DMF.

V. B. Copy to Applicant, Sponsor, or Other Holder

The holder should also send a copy of the letter of authorization to the affected applicant, sponsor, or other holder who is authorized to incorporate by reference the specific information contained in the DMF. include a copy of the DMF holder's letter of authorization in the application.

VI. PROCESSING AND REVIEWING POLICIES

VI. A. Policies Related to Processing Drug Master Files

VI. A.1. Public availability of the information and data in a DMF is determined under 21 CFR Part 20, 21 CFR 314.420(e), and 21 CFR 314.430.

VI. A.2. An original DMF submission will be examined on receipt to determine whether it meets minimum requirements for format and content. If the submission is administratively acceptable, FDA will acknowledge its receipt and assign it a DMF number.

If the submission is administratively incomplete or inadequate, it will be returned to the submitter with a letter of explanation from the Drug Master File Staff, and it will not be assigned a DMF number.

VI. B. Drug Master File Review

A DMF IS NEVER APPROVED OR DISAPPROVED.

The agency will review information in a DMF only when an IND sponsor, an applicant for an NDA, ANDA, or Export Application, or another DMF holder incorporates material in the DMF by reference. As noted, the incorporation by reference must be accompanied by a copy of the DMF holder's letter of authorization.

If FDA reviewers find deficiencies in the information provided in a DMF, a letter describing the deficiencies is sent to the DMF holder. At the same time, FDA will notify the person who relies on the information in the deficient DMF that additional information is needed in the supporting DMF. The general subject of the deficiency is identified, but details of the deficiency are disclosed only to the DMF holder. When the holder submits the requested information to the DMF in response to the agency's deficiency letter, the holder should also send a copy of the accompanying transmittal letter to the affected persons relying on the DMF and to the FDA reviewing division that identified the deficiencies. The transmittal letter will provide notice that the deficiencies have been addressed.

VII. HOLDER OBLIGATIONS

Any change or addition, including a change in authorization related to specific customers, should be submitted in duplicate and adequately cross referenced to previous submission(s). The reference should include the date(s), volume(s), section(s), and/or page number(s) affected.

VII. A. Notice Required for Changes to a Drug Master File

A holder must notify each affected applicant or sponsor who has referenced its DMF of any pertinent change in the DMF (21 CFR 314. 420(c)). Notice should be provided well before making the change in order to permit the sponsor/applicant to supplement or amend any affected application(s) as needed.

VII. B. Listing of Persons Authorized To Refer to a Drug Master File

VII. B.1.

A DMF is required to contain a complete list of persons authorized to incorporate information in the DMF The holder should update the list in the annual update. The updated list should contain the holder's name, DMF number, and the date of the update. The update should identify by name (or code) the information that each person is authorized to incorporate and give the location of that information by date, volume, and page number.

VII. B.2.

Any person whose authorization has been withdrawn during the previous year should be identified under a suitable caption.

VII. B.3.

If the list is unchanged on the anniversary date, the DMF holder should also submit a statement that the list is current.

VII. C. Annual Update

The holder should provide an annual report on the anniversary date of the original submission. This report should contain the required list as described in B.1., and should also identify all changes and additional information incorporated into the DMF since the previous annual report on the subject matter of the DMF. If the subject matter of the DMF is unchanged, the DMF holder should provide a statement that the subject matter of the DMF is current.

Failure to update or to assure FDA annually that previously submitted material and lists in the DMF remain current can cause delays in FDA review of a pending IND, NDA, ANDA, Export Application, or any amendment or supplement to such application; and FDA can initiate procedures for closure of the DMF (see Section IX).

VII. D. Appointment of an Agent

When an agent is appointed, the holder should submit a signed letter of appointment to the DMF giving the agent's name, address, and scope of responsibility (administrative and/or scientific). Domestic DMF holders do not need to appoint an agent or representative, although foreign DMF holders are encouraged to engage a U.S. agent.

VII. E. Transfer of Ownership

To transfer ownership of a DMF to another party, the holder should so notify FDA and authorized persons in writing. The letter should include the following:

1. Name of transferee

2. Address of transferee

3. Name of responsible official of transferee

4. Effective date of transfer

5. Signature of the transferring official

6. Typewritten name and title of the transferring official.

The new holder should submit a letter of acceptance of the transfer and an update of the information contained in the DMF, where appropriate. Any change relating to the new ownership (e.g., plant location and methods) should be included.

VIII. MAJOR REORGANIZATION OF A DRUG MASTER FILE

A holder who plans a major reorganization of a DMF is encouraged to submit a detailed plan of the proposed changes and request its review by the Drug Master File Staff. The staff should be given sufficient time to comment and provide suggestions before a major reorganization is undertaken.

IX. CLOSURE OF A DRUG MASTER FILE

A holder who wishes to close a DMF should submit a request to the Drug Master File Staff stating the reason for the closure. See Section IV.D.5.a for the address.

The request should include a statement that the holder's obligations as detailed in Section VII have been fulfilled.

The Agency may close a DMF that does not contain an annual update of persons authorized to incorporate information in the DMF by reference and a list of changes made since the previous annual report. The holder will be notified of FDA's intent to close the DMF.

5.9 SUBMISSIONS OF US FDA

> Submit complete dossiers by understanding the critical elements of US INDs and NDAs

> Meet the data requirements for INDs and NDAs

> Communicate better with the FDA by knowing the organizational structure of the Agency and the interactions within the agency

> Work your way through the laws and regulations governing the registration of prescription drugs in the US

> Know how to obtain information from the FDA

> Understand the logistics of the sponsor-FDA interactions

> Achieve faster drug registration in the US and be 'first, to market' to win market share

> Clarify the needs, expectations and regulatory requirements of the FDA for the drug registration dossier

> Prepare successful Investigational New Drug Applications (INDs) & New Drug Applications (NDA).

REVIEW QUESTIONS

ESSAY QUESTIONS

1. Explain the details of CDSCO and give its functions.

2. Write about various drug regulatory agencies?

3. Give a detail description on Australian TGA.

4. Give introduction to NDA & ANDA submission of US FDA.

5 . a. Write about suplimentary new drug application?

b. Describe treatment of IND for an orphan drug?

SHORT QUESTIONS

1. Canadian HPFBI

2. NDA

3. USFDA

Chapter 6

QUALITY ASSURANCE

6.1 INTRODUCTION

Quality Assurance. The ISO definition reads: *"the assembly of all planned and systematic actions necessary to provide adequate confidence that a product, process, or service will satisfy given quality requirements."* The result of these actions aimed at the production of quality, should ideally be checked by someone independent of the work: the Quality Assurance Officer. If no QA officer is available, then usually the Head of Laboratory performs this job as part of his quality management task. In case of special projects, customers may require special quality assurance measures or a Quality Plan.

Planned activities designed to ensure that the quality control activities are being properly implemented.

Quality assurance is the hart and the soul of quality control. Quality assurance consists of guarantening that a consumer can purchase a prduct with confidence and enjoy its satiafactory use for a long period. Quality assurance is the activity of providing the evidence needed to stablish confidence among all concerned that the quality function is effectively being followed.

Quality Assurance = Qaulity control + Good Manufacturing Practices.

6.2 THE PRINCIPLE OF QUALITY ASSURANCE

A company must practice quality assurance in order to guarantee and satisfy the customers and win their trust. Quality Assurance is achieved only if customer develops trust in the company itself, so that the consumer feel confident to purchase even new product form it.

To achive this the following principles must be followed:

➤ Adopt a 100% customer first approach ad obtain a firm grasp of consumers requirement.

➤ Hammer out a clear customer- First philosophy and ensure that everybody from the company president down is concerned with quality.

➤ Constantly rotate the quality cycle (The deming cycle) and never step improving quality.

➤ Producers and marketers are responsible for Quality Assurance.

➤ Follow " the next process is your customer"

Quality Assurance System Organization

The quality Assurance System organization can be represented as

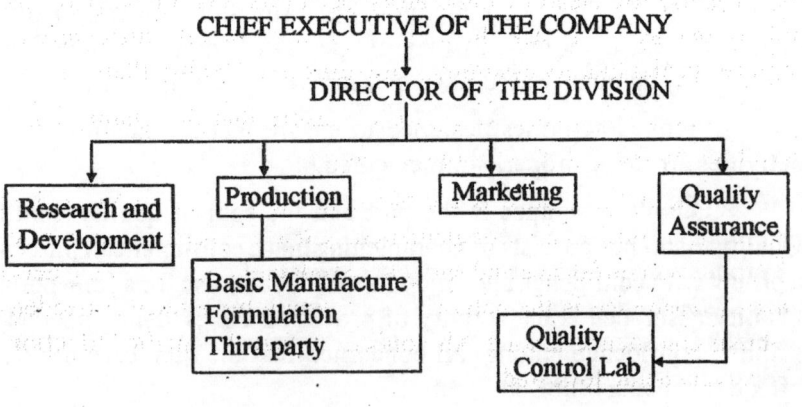

Fig.1: Responsibilities Of Quality Assurance

➤ Assurance that the adopted policies by a company are followed.

➤ Severs as contact with regulatory agencies.

➤ Final authority for product acceptance or rejection.

➤ Identifies and prepare the necessary standard operating procedures relative to the control of quality.

➤ During final product release, it must be determined that the product meets all the applicable specifications and that it was manufactured according to internal standards and the GMP's

➤ Major responsibility is a quality monitoring or audit function. Current and correct procedures, by properly trained operator is checked by quality assurance.

6.3 MANUFACTURING CONTROL

Although the scope and structure of the manufacturing control operation differs appreciably from company to company, it is possible to highlight their common element. The production planning department issues the formula and manufacturing worksheets bearing an identification number, title of product and the names and the quantities for all ingredients, together with the complete description of the procedures to be the followed, the precaution to be taken, the equipment to be used, the lot sizes to be processed and the suitable in- process controls to be undertaken. Material tickets for each raw material are written and issued by the production department to the department of material stores, where the orders are filled and verified. After the materials have been sent to the production department and checked similarly, the pattern of control takes shape as production proceeds. The addition of raw materials to the batch is verified and countersigned by a qualified person. Notation is made on the manufacturing worksheet of the identifying number of each ingredients it is performed. An appropriate label is attached to identify its contents and to ensure that the in-process stage is properly designated. Any deviations from standard operating conditions, no matter how small, should be reported to both production and control personnel responsible for the products.

The in-process checking during manufacturing plays an important role in the auditing of the quality of the product at various stages of production. Duties of the auditor or the control inspector consist of checking, enforcing, and reviewing procedures and suggesting the change for upgrading the procedures when necessary. The primary objective of an IPQC system is to monitor all the features of a product that may affect its quality and to prevent errors during processing. Only the most commonly practiced methods for parenterals, and semisolid preparations (ointments, creams and lotions) are briefly described.

For parenteral products, the in-process quality controls are

1. Checking the bulk solutions, before filling, for drug content, pH, color, clarity and completeness of solutions.

2. Checking of the filled volume of liquids or the filled weight of sterile powders for injection in the final containers at predetermined intervals during filling.

3. Testing for leakage of flame-sealed ampoules.

4. Subjecting the product to physical examination (visual or mechanically) for appearance, clarity and particulate contamination.

5. Examinating the product for sterility indicator placed in various areas of the sterilizer for each sterilization operation.

6. Submitting the product for sterility testing or other predetermined biologic tests to establish the safety and other parameters of the products.

The in-process quality controls for solid dosage forms are

1. Determining the drug content of the formulation

2. Checking the weight variation for tablet and capsules at pre determined intervals during manufacturing

3. Checking the disintegration and/or dissolution time, hardness and friability of the tablets atleast during the beginning, middle and

the end of production or at prescribed intervals during manufacturing.

4. Testing soluble tablets for compliance with solution time requirements and

5. Examining products by line inspection or other equally suitable means or removing the defective units prior to package.

For semisolid preparations, the following in process controls are available

1. Checking for uniformity and homogeneity of drug content prior to the filling operations

2. Determining the particle size of the preparation when appropriate

3. Checking the appearance, viscosity, specific gravity, sediment volume and other physical parameters at prescribed intervals.

4. Testing for filling weight during the filling operations and

5. Testing for leakage on the finished jars or tubes.

At the completion of the manufacturing process as well as in-process stages, actual yields are checked against theoretic value, and the representative samples are withdrawn for laboratory testing by the control inspector according to the predetermined sampling plan. The operators actively performing the process, their supervisors and the control inspector must all verify that the entire operation was accomplished in the prescribed manner. Occasionally materials in bulk storage are sampled at random and are examined to determine that no detectable change has taken place and that the batch is satisfactory for final packaging.

The batch production records and other needed documents are then delivered to the quality control office, together with the withdrawn samples of the products. These records and test results are reviewed for conformance to specifications and CGMP. The bulk finished products are held in quarantine until they are released for packing by quality control personnel.

6.4 CONTROL AND ASSURANCE OF MANUFACTURING PRACTICES

The factory inspection provision of the 1962 amendments to the food, drug and cosmetic act empowered the FDA to inspect drug manufacturing sites with compliance with accepted standards of operations, practices and sanitation. The law recognizes that the Current Good Manufacturing Practices (cGMP) with the attendant quality control procedure are paramount to the production of quality products. As a result, the FDA has required pharmaceutical s manufacturers to commit themselves to a method of manufacturing and quality assurance for each product. The manufacturer should have performed sufficient control test to permit an evaluation of adequacy of the manufacturing, processing and packaging operation.

The first cGMP regulation where issued in 1963 one year after the enactment of the 1962 Kefauver- Harris Drug Amendments. The word 'current' in referring to cGMP, suggests that they are dynamic, and the regulatory agencies constantly updates and maintains them in relation to the current state of the art and science of drug manufacturing practices of the industries. The next revision took place in 1978, and these are in effect at present.

The successful application of cGMP is complex but possible if systems governing the various phages of personnel, equipment, buildings, control records and production procedures are at the state of proper planning and control. It should be kept in mind that cGMP is an aid and by no means a substitute for a good total quality assurance program.

Personnel

One criterion for a successful quality assurance program is the encouragement of quality consciousness in the personnel of the entire company. Proper selection, training and motivation of production, packaging and control personnel are vital to produce quality pharmaceuticals consistently. The degree to which the desired quality for the product is attainable is proportional to the attitudes or desires of the individual working in production, packaging and control. By building a sense of pride in performance and showing the importance of the contributions of these individuals in producing products that could be lifesaving, the risk of errors can be minimized. In reality, this is the zero-defect concept, which operates through prevention rather than detection of the mistakes by properly directing and motivating personnel. Quality work and products result from this approach.

It is essential that qualified personnel be employed to supervise the formulation, processing, sampling, testing, packaging and labeling of the drug product, and that competent staff be placed in charge of the maintenance of machinery, equipment and sanitation. The qualified personnel are the person who by virtue of education training and experience has the knowledge and ability to execute the technologic assignments. The key personnel involved in the manufacture and control of the drug should assume the responsibility of assuring that the drug and dosage form they are handling have the desired characteristics. The responsibility for keeping manufacturing process within the cGMP regulation of FDC Act must be delegated to the people directly involved with the various aspects of the process and their immediate supervisor are required to provide the necessary direction and control of the operation and be available at all times in case a question or a problem arises. The operating personnel should have the necessary authority to sign the manufacturing documents for each process for which they are responsible. The document is then countersigned by the supervisor. The signature and endorsement should appear on the proper worksheet at the completion of a production operation.

Equipment and Buildings

Equipment and Building used in the manufacture, processing, packaging, labeling, storage, or control of the drug should be of suitable design, size, construction, and location, and should be maintained in clean a clean and orderly manner.

The building should provide adequate space for the orderly placement of materials and equipment to minimize any risks of mixps or cross contamination between the drugs, excipients, packaging and labeling from the time the materials are received to the time the products are released. Adequate lighting, ventilation, dust control, temperature and humidity should also be provided. To avoid conditions unfavorable to the integrity and safety of the product, other considerations may be required for particular operations and products, such as bacteriologic controls for preventing microbial contamination, for sanitizing work areas for parenteral preparations and for preventing the dissemination of microorganisms from one area to another or from previous manufacturing operations.

The desired characteristics of equipment for producing quality products are numerous and they differ from machine to machine. However, the equipment should be of suitable size, accuracy and reproducibility. Their surfaces should be inert, non reactive, non absorptive and non additive so that the identity, purity and quality of the drug substance and other components are not affected to any significant extent. The equipment should be constructed to facilitate adjustment, cleaning and maintenance to assure the precision, reliability, and uniformity of the process and product, and to assure the exclusion of contaminants from previous and current manufacturing and packaging operations.

Control of records

The records, such as master formula and batch production records, should be prepared and maintained in accordance with established procedures.

Master formula record

Master formula record for each product should be prepared, endorsed, and dated by the competent and responsible individual and should be independently checked, endorsed and dated by another competent and responsible individual. The information contained in the records should be provided in the format and language that will not be misinterpreted by the operating personnel and the supervisor, to assure that the each batch of product can be identically reproduced.

Although the content and format may differ from product to product, the master formula record shall include the following information:

1. The name of the product, a description of the dosage form, and its strength.

2. The complete list of ingredients, designated by whole names and codes sufficiently specific to indicate any special characteristic.

3. The quantity by weight or volume of each ingredient, regardless of whether it appears in the finished product. If variations in the quantity of a particular ingredient are permitted, as is sometimes necessary in the preparation of the dosage form, an adequate statement should be provided in the record.

4. The standards or specifications of each ingredient used in the product.

5. An appropriate statement concerning any calculated excess of an ingredient.

6. Appropriate statement of the theoretical yield at various stages and the termination of the processing.

7. Manufacturing and control instructions, specifications, precautions and special notations to be followed.

8. A detailed descriptions of the closures, containers, labeling, packaging and other finishing materials.

Batch Production Records

Batch production records should be prepared, maintained and controlled for each batch of products. In general they should be retained for a period of approximately five years after distribution has been completed. The batch production record shall contain an accurate reproduction of the manufacturing formula, procedure and product specifications from the correct master formula procedure to be used in the production of batch of product. These batch records are then sent to each of the departments involved in the production, packaging and control of the product. The records include dates, specific dates or identifications numbers of each ingredient employed, weights or measures of components and products in the course of processings, results of in-process and control testing, and the endorsement of the individual performing and supervising each step of the operation.

In addition, a lot number is assigned that permits the identification of all procedure perform on the lot and their results. These lot number appears on the label of the product these procedure facilitates a search for details of manufacture and control history of any particular product.

Control of production procedures

To ensure that the products have the intended characteristics of identity, strength, quality and purity, production and the related in-process quality control (IPQC) procedures should be rigidly followed as required by the master formula record or the batch production record. To a large extent, IPQC is concerned with providing accurate, specific and definite description of procedures to be employed from the receipts of the raw material to the release of the finished dosage forms.

It is a planned system

➢ To identify the materials, equipment, processes, and operators;

➢ To enforce the flow of manufacturing and packaging operations according to the established rules and practices.

➢ To minimize human error or to detect the error if and when it does occur.

➢ To pinpoint the responsibility to the personnel involved in each unit operation of the entire process.

In general the in-process control procedures are usually rapid and simple tests or inspections that are performed when the manufacturing of a product batch is in process. They are used to detect variations from the tolerance limit of the product so that prompt and corrective action can be taken. The in-process control procedures and tests should be openly discussed, experimentally justified, written in detail, properly explained, and in particular, rigidly enforced once they are established.

The production procedures are subdivided into

➢ Manufacturing control

➢ Packaging control

Packaging control

At sometimes at the manufacture of a product is completed; a packaging record bearing an identification number is issued to the packaging section. This record specifies the packaging materials to be used, operations to be performed and the quantity to be packaged. Simultaneously, requisitions are issued for the products to be packed and for the packaging and printed materials, such as labels, containers, inserts, brochures, cartons, and shipping cases.

The packaging operation unites the product, container and labels to form a single finished unit. Not only must individual package components be correct, but they must also be assembled correctly. Prior to the start of packaging operation, the control inspector and packaging supervisor must check and verify the line to ensure that it has been thoroughly been cleaned and that all materials from the previous packaging have been completely removed. In addition, various species of packaging equipment are stripped down, cleaned, and examined when an order is finished. The bulk of the product and each of the packaging components should be checked, endorsed and dated by qualified packing personnel with the cooperation of control inspector. In practice, the exact number of labels required for a batch, including a small excess, should be delivered to the labeling area after careful and meticulous inspection of each label.

In the packaging area a large group of people work on several different products simultaneously, using high-speed packaging equipment. Therefore, the operation should be performed with adequate physical segregation of products. Dosage forms of similar color, size, and shape should not be scheduled consecutively on a line. Tablets of similar shape should not be scheduled on the neighboring packaging lines at the same time, even though the size or color may be dissimilar. Proper on-line inspection should be made during the packaging operation to insure absence of foreign drugs and labels, adequacy of the containers and closures, and accuracy of labeling. Proper reconciliation and disposition of the unused and wasted labels should occur at the end of the packaging operations. The yield must be justified against the theory represented by the batch size of the starting material. Suitable and reasonable procedures should be established for action to be taken when an unexplained discrepancy exists between the number of labels issued and the number accounted for on the finished products. The common approach is for key personnel to prevent distribution of the batch in question, and of other batches of products that were packaged during the same period of time, until a satisfactory explanation can be obtained for a discrepancy.

Packaging materials control

The USP defines the container closure system as that device that holds the drug and is or may be in direct contact with the drug. The immediate container is that which is in direct contact with the drug at all times. The closure is a part of the container.

Packaging materials should not interact physically or chemically with the finished product to alter the strength, quality, or purity beyond specified requirements. The compendium provides specifications and tests procedures for light resistance: well closed, tightly closed, and four different types of glass containers.

Specifications and test methods are designed for containers on the basis of tests performed on the product in the container. The following features are to be considered in developing container specifications:

➤ Properties of container tightness

➤ Moisture and vapor tightness regardless of container construction.

➤ Toxicity and chemical/physical characteristics of materials needed in container construction

➤ Physical or chemical changes of container upon prolonged contact with product.

➤ Compatibility between container and product

Good manufacturing practices require that stability data be submitted for the finished dosage form of drug in the container closure system in which it is to be marketed.

Label control

Production control issues of packaging forms that carries

> ➤ the name of the product

> ➤ item number

> ➤ lot number

> ➤ number of labels, inserts and packaging materials to be used

> ➤ Operations to be performed and the quantity to be packaged.

A copy of this form is sent to the supervisor of label control, who intern counts out the required number of labels. Since labels may be spoiled during the packaging operations a definite number in excess of that actually required is usually issued; however, all labels must be accounted for at the end of operation, and unused labels must be accounted for before their destruction.

If the lot number and expiration date of the product are not going to be printed directly on the line, the labels are run through a printing machine which imprint the lot number and the expiration date. The labels are recounted and placed in a separate container with proper identification for further transfer to the packing department. The packaging department then requests, according to the packaging form, the product to be packaged, along with all packaging components, such as labels, inserts, bottles, vials, ampoules, stoppers, caps, seals, cartons and shipping cases. Quality assurance personnel inspects and verifies all packaging components and equipment to be used for the packaging operations to ensure that it has the proper identification, that the line has been thoroughly cleaned, and that all materials from the previous packaging operation have been completely removed. Proper reconciliation and disposition of the unused and wasted labels should occur at the end of the packaging operations.

Quality Assurance during Packaging Operations

If the quality control laboratory analysis confirms that the product complies with specification, and if the quality assurance audit indicates that manufacturing operations are satisfactory, the bulk product is released to the packaging department, and the production control is notified. Packaging operations should be performed with adequate physical segregation from product to product. Quality assurance personnel should periodically inspect the packaging lines and should check filled and labeled containers for compliance with return specification. Some packaging operation, especially those using high-speed equipment, are fitted with automated testing equipment to check each container for fill and label placement. Alternatively, an operator may visually inspect all packages fed into the final cartons. Quality assurance should perform an independent inspection and select finished preservation samples at random from each lot. The preservation samples should consists of atleast twice the quantity necessary to perform all tests required to determine whether the product meets its established specification. These preservation samples should be retained for atleast one year after the expiration date and should be stored their original package under conditions consistent with product labeling.

Quality assurance personnel should also select an appropriate size sample of the finished package product and send it to the analytic control laboratory for final testing.

Auditing

Good manufacturing practice requires that the manufacturing process be adequately documented throughout all stages of the operations. The history of all tasks, including the starting materials, equipments used, personnel involved in production and control until completed packaging is complete, should be recorded. The areas of record keeping include:

➤ Individual components, raw materials, and packaging materials. Master formula and procedure.

➤ Batch production.

➤ Packaging and labeling operations.

➤ Laboratory in-process and finished control testing.

➢ Proper signing and dating by atleast two individuals independently for each operation in the proper spaces.

➢ Reconciliations of the materials supplied with accounts of tablets produced, taking into account allowable loss limits.

Before releasing the product for distribution quality assurance should evaluate the batch records of all in-process tests and controls and of all tests of the final product to determine whether they confirm to specifications.

Packaging Control

Once pharmaceutical products have been manufactured, and prior to their despatch, they need to be stored within a carefully controlled storage environment. Within the warehouse, temperature and humidity levels must not exceed specified limits, and details of actual variations in these key parameters must be logged in order to meet FDA guidelines. This may be achieved by monitoring temperature and humidity sensors continuously using a network of highly accurate Eurotherm graphical recorders. These sophisticated instruments, supported by powerful data display and analysis software, can record and archive data in an encrypted tamper-proof format, allowing the system to support FDA validation and in particular 21 CFR Part 11 compliance. In a typical installation, which would be required to monitor environmental storage conditions throughout several warehouses, each warehouse would be monitored by a multi-channel Eurotherm graphical recorder, such as the Model 6180V. This instrument, continuously measuring the signals from combined temperature and humidity probes sited at key points within the warehouse, are connected within an Ethernet LAN to a centrally located secure server for long term data storage and supervisory control purposes.

Each data recorder is capable of monitoring up to 48 combined temperature and humidity sensors within each warehouse, and providing a local screen display of both current and recent conditions as well transmitting this information to remote supervisory PCs. The recorders can flag 'Alert' and 'Excursion' alarms if warehouse conditions go outside acceptable values, as well as providing alarm summary and alarm history reports when required. Hardwired alarm notification can also be provided to local control or security centres. These recorders are capable of automatically calculating Mean Kinetic Temperature (MKT), and the touch screen interface on each instrument allows individual sensors to be removed from the MKT calculation during calibration. Pre-configured reports can be generated for each warehouse. Since such systems will be fully validated to FDA 21 CFR part 11 compliance standards, they need to be developed using a formal project lifecycle approach. Operation will be password protected, with individual user accounts, inactivity timeout, password expiry, and automatic audit trail of operator actions built-in as standard. Separate, high-integrity data collection will be arranged for each warehouse, usually supported by uninterruptible power supplies for each recorder. This allows secure local storage of process data, alarm and event data, and audit trail messages. Automatic archiving of data over the local Ethernet network to a secure server PC is scheduled on a regular basis, allowing site executives to retrieve key data for off-line viewing and report generation.

A typical sensor signal will be brought into each local graphic recorder as a 4-20mA signal. By calculating a group average of all temperature and humidity readings in the warehouse, alerts and excursion alarms may be set up should readings stray outside acceptable limits. In order to permit calculation of mean kinetic temperature (MKT) for reports, each channel will have an associated daily maximum and minimum value, which is then grouped and averaged for all sensors in the warehouse. Individual sensors can be automatically removed from the MKT calculation (for example, when selected for calibration or on a fault condition) by holding the maximum and minimum channels at the last 'good' value. Systems such as these would normally utilise sophisticated software to ensure that each recorder is in constant communication with the central supervisory PC, and that reports are automatically generated and archived on a regular basis. The Eurotherm Bridge package is designed specifically for this purpose, and has a proven track record with the Eurotherm Series of graphical recorders. The software will allow UHH files of current data and alarms/recent history to be stored locally in flash memory and then automatically archived at set intervals to the filing system on the central control point (primary server).

This will be done in an encrypted, tamper proof format.

Detailed reports, usually in Excel format, may be generated at any time, and secondary server details can also be set up, allowing each recorder to archive to the secondary server should the primary become unavailable.

6.5 QUALITY CONTROL

The main objective of the quality control programme is to ensure the supply of a standard product to customer so as to get his satisfaction. The QC programme also assure the accuracy and precision as well as the reliability of the claim given on the label. The quality control programme helps to get the desired raw materials, intermediates of packing materials, which would ultimately result in the final product of the desired standard.

Some Misunderstandings about Quality Control

- QC costs money.
- QC means making standards.
- QC consists of tightening up inspection.
- QC is statistics.
- QC is nothing to do with administration department
- QC is nothing to do with me.
- QC is something the QC section does.
- We are making profit at the moment, so we don't need anything like QC.

The Benefits of Quality Control

- Quality is raised, the number of defective products decreases
- Costs decrease
- Products can be sold at higher prices.

- Reliability increased confidence in the products improves, and customers trust is obtained.

- Productivity increase.

- Wasteful work disappears, rework decreases and efficiency improves

- Inspection and testing costs decrease.

- Quality become more uniform and the number of complaints decrease

- Employee's humanity is respected, personnel development becomes possible and workplaces become more cheerful.

- Talent-spotting becomes possible, and people are able to exercise their full capacitites.

- People become able to talk frankly and openly.

- Decision making is speeded up and policy deployment and management by objectives improve.

- The corporate culture is improved.

- The company becomes trusted.

- New-Product development speeds up and improves. Products of world beating quality can be made

6.6 IDEAL QUALITY CONTROL LAB

Quality control lab should be suitably designed, equipped and maintained to suit the activities to be carried out in them. There should be sufficient space for carrying out all the tests and for non-laboratory requirements such as administration offices, storage areas for chemicals, instrument spaces, records and reserve samples of products and applicable computer areas.

An ideal lab should possess:

➤ Analytical laboratory for carrying out the chemical test, instrument room, flame proof areas rooms for report writing.

➤ Microbiological laboratories, microbiological array areas, and work areas for enviorment-monitoring microbiological tests.

➤ Sterility testing laboratories with changing rooms.

➤ Packaging material testing areas.

➤ Waste areas.

➤ Storage areas.

➤ Biological testing room if required.

Chemical biological and microbiological laboratories should be separated from each other and from manufacturing areas. Animal houses should be well isolated.

10% of total laboratories areas should be set aside for storage of chemicals glassware, solvent and gas cylinders. Sensitive instruments should be kept away from vibrations, excessive humidity, fumes etc.

Particular attention should be paid to the arrangements for the safe storage of waste materials awaiting disposal. For operations involving fume or fuming liquids. Fume cupboard should be provided. The cupboard for flammable solvent operation should be separate.

Floors should be stain resistant and solvent resistant the floor to wall and wall to ceiling points should be coined and walls should be smooth and non-absorbent.

Bench levels should suit the type of equipment placed on them, and it should be provided with water, gas, vaccum.

Drainage should be of heavy duty plastics, sinks of ceramic or stainless steel.

Voltage stabilizer for voltage fluctuation, Illumination of work area must be efficient.

The laboratories should have sufficient equipment and instrumentation to carry out all the tests required for quality control and for providing analytical services to the product development department.

The method of calibration and acceptance criteria for the results of the calibration tests must be recorded in form of a SOP, each item of equipment.

Quality control lab should posses skilled staff. They must be trained in laboratory techniques including classical chemical analysis, instrumental techniques and microbiological methods. Personnel must also be trained in the principles of GMP.

REVIEW QUESTIONS

1.   a. Write the concept of quality assurance?

b. Explain about the raw material quality assurance monograph?

2.   Write the quality assurance activities related to ware house control and manufacturing control?

3.   a. Write the sources and control of quality variation?

b. Write the quality assurance activities related to packaging control?

4.   Write short notes on the following

a.   Quality control documents

b.   Quality audit

c.   Batch release document

Chapter 7

GOOD MANUFACTURING PRACTICES

7.1 INTRODUCTION

Good Manufacturing Practice (GMP) is that part of Quality Assurance which ensures that products are consistently produced and controlled to appropriate quality standards and involves all facets of manufacturing, warehouse, production, quality control testing, engineering and personal hygiene of staff.

GMP is practiced by law worldwide following different guidelines like 21 CFR- part 210 and 211 in USA, EUGMP in Europe and WHOGMP in over 100 member countries. WHO has defined Good Manufacturing Practice as "GMP is a part of quality assurance, which ensures that products are consistently produced and controlled to the quality standards appropriate to their intended use and as required by the marketing authorization". In India, GMP was enacted as Schedule M to Drug and Cosmetics Rules in 1988 and upgraded in 2003 as revised Schedule M.

Significance of Good Manufacturing Practice in Pharmaceutical Industry

Following good manufacturing practice are intended in Pharmaceutical Industry to assure that:

- All the raw materials used in the manufacture process are of standard quality and are free from contamination.
- All the equipments used in the manufacture process are qualified.

- All manufacturing operations are carried out under the supervision of technical staff approved by the licensing authority.

- Adequate controls on starting materials, intermediate products, and bulk products and other in process controls, calibrations and validations are carried out.

- All the In-process materials are tested for identity, strength, quality and purity as appropriate and approved or rejected by the quality control unit, during production process.

- All packaging materials to be used are checked on delivery to the packaging department for quantity, identity & conformity with the packaging instructions.

- No batch of the product shall be released for the sale or supply until the authorized persons that it is in accordance with the requirements of the standards laid down have certified it.

- Records for distribution are maintained in such a manner that finished batch of a product can be traced to the retail level to facilitate prompt and complete recall of the batch, if and when necessary.

7.2 GMP IN INDIA

Even though Indian medical system was one of the oldest, collective efforts to practice GMPs as it was defined in other advanced countries was not there until 1988, when Government of India amended the Drugs & Cosmetics Rules, 1945 vide G.S.R. 735 (E) dated 24 June 1988 first Schedule M-Good Manufacturing Practices and Requirement of Premises, Plant and Equipment was published. The guidelines have been more elaborated and made more in line with expectations of international practices of GMPs. The1988 guidelines are upgraded in 2003 as revised Schedule M. Revised section has given new dimension and meanings to GMP, it is more popularly known as schedule M (Rule 71, 74, 76 and 78) good manufacturing practices and requirements of premises, plant and equipment for pharmaceutical products.

GOOD MANUFACTURING PRACTICES AND REQUIREMENTS OF PREMISES, PLANT AND EQUIPMENT FOR PHARMACEUTICAL PRODUCTS

[SCHEDULE M]

(Rules 71, 74, 76, and 78)

Schedule M Part	Deal with provision
Part I	Good manufacturing practices for premises and materials
Part I - A	Specific requirement for manufacturer of sterile products, parenteral and Sterile ophthalmic preparations
Part I - B	Specific requirement for manufacturer of oral solid dosage form(Tablets and capsules)
Part I - C	Specific requirement for manufacturer of oral liquid dosage form (Syrups, Elixirs, Emulsions and Suspensions)
Part I - D	Specific requirement for manufacturer of topical products i.e. external preparations (creams, emulsion, lotion, solutions, dusting powders)
Part I - E	Specific requirement for manufacturer of Meter dose Inhaler
Part I - F	Specific requirement of premises, Plant and materials for manufacturer of Active Pharmaceutical Ingredient(Bulk drugs)
Part II	Requirements of Plants and Equipments

PART I

7.3 GOOD MANUFACTURING PRACTICES FOR PREMISES AND MATERIALS

1.GENERAL REQUIREMENTS

1.1 Location and surroundings

The factory building(s) for manufacture of drugs shall be so situated and shall have such measures as to avoid risk of contamination from external environment including open sewage, drain, public lavatory or any factory which produces disagreeable or obnoxious, odor, fumes, excessive soot, dust, smoke, chemical or biological emissions.

1.2 Buildings and premises

The building(s) used for the factory shall be designed, constructed, adapted and maintained to suit the manufacturing operations so as to permit production of drugs under hygienic conditions. The premises used for manufacturing, processing, warehousing, and packaging, labeling and testing purposes shall be compatible with other drug manufacturing operations that may be carried out in the same or adjacent area / section. Adequate space shall be provided to avoid mix-ups and cross-contamination.

Interior surface (walls, floors, and ceilings) shall be smooth and free from cracks, and permit easy cleaning, Painting and disinfections. The production and dispensing areas shall be well lighted, effectively ventilated, with air control facilities and may have proper Air handling units (wherever applicable) to maintain conditions including temperature and, wherever necessary, humidity, as defined for the relevant product.

1.3 Water system

There shall be validated system for treatment of water drawn from own or any other source to render it potable in accordance with standards specified by the Bureau of Indian Standards or local municipality, as the case may be, so as to produce purified water conforming to pharmacopoeial specification.

1.4 Disposal of waste

The disposal of swage and effluents (solid, liquid and gas) from the manufactory shall be in conformity with the requirements of Environment pollution control Board.

2. WAREHOUSING AREA

Adequate areas shall be designed to allow sufficient and orderly warehousing of various categories of materials and products like starting and packaging materials intermediates bulk and finished products, products in quarantine released, rejected, returned or recalled machine and equipment spare parts and change items.

Receiving and dispatch bays shall protect materials and products from adverse weather conditions. Highly hazardous, poisonous and explosive materials such as narcotics, psychotropic drugs and substances presenting potential risks of abuse, fire or explosion, shall be stored in safe and secure Areas. Printed packaging material shall be stored in safe, separate and secure areas.

Regular checks shall be made to ensure adequate steps are taken against spillage, breakage and leakage of containers.

3. PRODUCTION AREA

The production area shall be designed to allow the production preferably in uni-flow and with logical sequence of operations. Working and in process space shall be adequate to permit orderly and logical positioning of equipment and materials and movement of personnel to avoid cross-contamination and to minimize risk of omission or wrong application of any of manufacturing and control measures. Service lines shall preferably be identified by colors and the nature of the supply and direction of the flow shall be marked/ indicated.

4. ANCILLARY AREAS

Rest and refreshment rooms shall be separate from other areas. Facilities for changing storing clothes and for washing and toilet purposes shall be easily accessible and adequate for the number of users. Tools and spare parts for use in sterile areas shall be disinfected before these are carried inside the production areas. Areas housing animals shall be isolated from other areas.

5. QUALITY CONTROL AREA

Quality-Control Laboratories shall be independent of the production areas. Separate areas shall be provided each for physicochemical, biological, microbiological or radio-isotope analysis. Separate instrument room with adequate area shall be provided for sensitive and sophisticated instruments employed for analysis. Sufficient and suitable storage space shall be provided for test samples, retained samples, reference standards, reagents and records.

6. PERSONNEL

The manufacture shall he conducted under the direct supervision of competent technical staff with prescribed qualifications and practical experience in the relevant dosage form and/or active pharmaceutical products. The head of the Quality Control Laboratory shall be independent of the manufacturing unit. The testing shall be conducted-under the direct supervision of competent technical staff who shall be whole time employees of the licensee. Personnel for Quality Assurance and Quality Control operations shall be suitably qualified and experienced. Number of personnel employed shall be adequate and in direct proportion to the work-load.

7. HEALTH, CLOTHING AND SANITATION OF WORKERS

Prior to employment, all personnel, shall undergo medical examination including eye examination, and shall be free from Tuberculosis, skin and other communicable or contagious diseases. Thereafter, they should be medically examined periodically, at least once a year. All persons, prior to and during employment, shall be trained in practices which ensure personnel hygiene. All employees shall be instructed to report about their illness or abnormal health condition to their immediate supervisor so that appropriate action can be taken. All personnel shall wear clean body coverings appropriate to their duties. Smoking, eating, drinking, chewing or keeping plants, food, drink and personal medicines shall not be permitted in production.

8. MANUFACTURING OPERATIONS AND CONTROLS

All manufacturing operations shall be carried out under the supervision of technical staff approved by the Licensing Authority. Each critical step in the process relating to the selection, weighing and measuring of raw material addition during various stages shall be performed by trained personnel under the direct personnel supervision of approved technical staff. The contents of all vessels and containers used in manufacture and storage during the various manufacturing stages shall be conspicuously labeled with the name of the product, batch no, batch size and stage of manufacture. Each label should be initialed and dated by the authorized technical staff. Products not prepared under aseptic conditions are required to be free from pathogens like *Salmonella, Escherichia coli, Pyocyanea* etc.

9. SANITATION IN THE MANUFACTURING PREMISES

The manufacturing premises shall be cleaned and maintained in an orderly manner, so that it is free from accumulated waste, dust, debits and other similar material. A validated cleaning procedure shall be maintained.

10. RAW MATERIALS

The licensee shall keep an inventory of all raw-materials to be used at any stage of manufacture of drugs and maintain records as per Schedule U. All incoming materials shall be quarantined immediately after receipt or processing. All materials shall he stored under appropriate conditions and in an orderly fashion to permit batch segregation and stock rotation by a 'first in/first expiry' - 'first-out' principle. All incoming materials shall he purchased from approved sources under valid purchase vouchers. There shall be adequate separate areas for materials "under test", "approved ", and "rejected" with arrangements and equipment to allow dry, clean and orderly placement of stored materials and products, wherever necessary under controlled temperature and humidity.

11. EQUIPMENT

Equipment shall he located, designed, constructed, adapted and maintained to suit the operations to be earned out. The layout and design of the equipment shall aim to minimize the risk of errors and permit effective cleaning and maintenance in order to avoid cross contamination, build-up of dust or dirt and, in general, any adverse effect on the quality of products. Balances and other measuring equipment of an appropriate range, accuracy and precision shall be available in the raw-material stores.

12. DOCUMENTATION AND RECORDS

Documentation is an essential part of the Quality assurance system and, as such, shall be related to all aspects of Good Manufacturing

Practices (GMP). Its aim is to define the specifications for all materials, method of manufacture and control, to ensure that all personnel concerned with manufacture know the information necessary to decide whether or not to release a batch or a drug for sale and-to provide an audit trail that shall permit investigation of the history of any suspected defective batch.

13. LABELS AND OTILER PRINTED MATERIALS

The printing shall be done in bright colours and in a legible manner. The label shall carry all the prescribed details about the product. Prior to release, all labels for containers, cartons and boxes and all circulars, inserts and leaflets shall be examined by the Quality Control Department of the licensee. Records of receipt of all labeling and packaging materials shall be maintained for each shipment received indicating receipt, control reference numbers and whether accepted or rejected. Unused coded and damaged labels and packaging materials shall he destroyed and recorded.

14. QUALITY ASSURANCE

The system of quality assurance appropriate to the manufacture of pharmaceutical products shall ensure that the pharmaceutical products are not released for sale or supplied before authorized persons have certified that each production batch has been produced and controlled in accordance with the requirements of the label claim and any other provisions relevant to production, control and release of pharmaceutical products.

15. SELF INSPECTION AND QUALITY AUDIT

The program shall he designed to detect "shortcomings in the implementation of Good Manufacturing Practice and to recommend the necessary corrective actions. Self-inspections shall be performed routinely and on specific, occasions, like when product recalls or repeated rejections occur or when an inspection by the licensing authorities is announced. The team responsible for self-inspection shall consist of personnel who can evaluate the implementation of Good Manufacturing Practice objectively, all recommendations for corrective action shall be implemented.

16. QUALITY CONTROL SYSTEM

Quality control shall be concerned with sampling specifications, testing, documentation, release procedures which ensure that the necessary and relevant tests are actually carried and that the materials are not released for use, nor products released for sale or supply until their quality has been judged to be satisfactory.

17. SPECIFICATIONS

Specifications for raw materials, packaging materials, containers , closures and for finished products shall comply with the pharmacopoeial requirements.

18. MASTER FORMULA RECORDS

Master Formula records shall be prepared and endorsed by the competent technical staff. i.e.. head of production and quality control.

The Master Formula shall include-

(a) The name of the product together with product reference code relating to its specifications

(b) The patent or proprietary name of the product along with the generic name, a description of the dosage form, strength, composition of the product and batch size

(c) Name, quantity, and reference number of all the starting materials to be used. Mention shall be made of any substance that may 'disappear' in the course of processing

(d) A statement of the expected final yield with the acceptable limits, and of relevant intermediate yields, where applicable

(e) A statement of the processing location and the principal equipment to be used

(f) The methods. or reference to the methods, to be used for preparing the critical equipment including cleaning, assembling, calibrating, sterilizing

(g) Detailed stepwise processing instructions and the time taken

(h)   The instructions for in-process controls with their limits

(i)   The requirements for storage conditions of the products, including the container, labelling and special storage conditions where applicable

(j)   Any special precautions to be observed

(k)   Packing details and specimen labels

19. PACKAGING RECORDS

There shall be authorize packaging instructions for each product, pack size and type. Upon completion of the packing and labeling operation reconciliation shall be made between number of labeling and packaging units issued, number of units labeled, packed and excess returned or destroyed. Any significant or unusual discrepancy in the numbers shall be carefully investigated before releasing the final batch.

20. BATCH PACKAGING RECORDS

A batch packaging record shall be kept for each batch or part batch processed. It shall be based on the relevant parts of the packaging instructions and the method of preparation of such records shall be designed to avoid transcription errors. Before any packaging operations begins, checks shall be made and recorded that the equipment and the work stations are clear of the previous products, documents or materials not required for the planned packaging operations, and that the equipment is clean and suitable for use.

21. BATCH PROCESSING RECORDS

The Batch processing Record shall include-

a)   The name of the product,

b)   The number of the batch being manufactured,

c)   Dates and time of commencement, of significant intermediate stages and of completion of production,

d)   Initials of the operator of different significant steps of production and where appropriate, of the person who checked each of these operations,

e) The batch number and/or analytical control number as well as the quantities of each starting material actually weighed,

f) Any relevant processing operation or event and major equipment used,

g) A record of the in-process controls and the initials of the person(s) carrying them out, and the results obtained,

h) The amount of product obtained after different and critical stages of manufacture (yield),

i) Comments or explanations for significant deviations from the expected yield limits shall be given,

j) Notes on special problems -including details, with signed authorization, for any deviation from the master formula,

k) Addition of any recovered or reprocessed material with reference to recovery or reprocessing stages.

22. STANDARD OPERATING PROCEDURES (SOPS) AND RECORDS, REGARDING

There shall be written Standard Operating Procedures and records for the receipt of each delivery of raw, primary and printed packaging material, for sampling, numbering of batch and for maintaince of analysis records.

23. REFERENCE SAMPLES

Each lot of every active ingredient in a quantity sufficient to carry out all the tests except sterility and pyrogens /Bacterial Endotoxin shall be retained for a period of 3 months after the date of expiry of the last batch produced from that active ingredient. Samples of finished formulations shall be stored in the same or simulated containers in which the drug has been actually marketed.

24. REPROCESSING AND RECOVERIES

Where reprocessing is necessary, written procedures shall be established and approved by the Quality Assurance Department that shall specify the conditions and limitations of repeating chemical reactions.

Such reprocessing shall be validated. Recovery of product residue may be carried out, if permitted, in the master production and control records by incorporating it in subsequent batches of the product.

25. DISTRIBUTION RECORDS

Prior to distribution or dispatch of given batch of a drug, it shall be ensured that the batch has been duly tested, approved and released by the quality control personnel. Records for distribution shall be maintained in a manner such that finished batch of a drug can be traced to the retail level to facilitate prompt and complete recall of the batch, if and when necessary.

26. VALIDATION AND PROCESS VALIDATION

Validation studies shall be an essential part of Good Manufacturing Practices and shall be conducted as per the pre-defined protocols. These shall include validation of processing, testing and cleaning procedures. A written report summarizing recorded results and conclusions shall be prepared, documented and maintained. Processes and procedures shall be established on the basis of validation study and undergo periodic revalidation to ensure that they remain capable of achieving the intended results. Critical processes shall be validated, prospectively or retrospectively.

27. PRODUCT RECALLS

A prompt and effective product recall system of defective products shall be devised for timely information of all concerned stockiest, wholesalers, suppliers, up to the retail level within the shortest period. There shall be an established written procedure in the form of Standard Operating Procedure for effective recall of products distributed by the licensee.

28. COMPLAINTS AND ADVERSE REACTIONS

All complaints there of concerning product quality shall be carefully reviewed and recorded according to written procedures. Each complaint shall be investigated/evaluated by the designated personnel of the company and records of investigation and remedial action taken thereof shall be maintained. Reports of serious adverse drug reactions resulting from the use of a drug along with comments and documents shall be forthwith reported to the concerned Licensing Authority.

29. SITE MASTER FILE

The licensee shall prepare a succinct document in the form of Site Master File containing specific and factual Good Manufacturing Practices about the production and/or control of pharmaceutical manufacturing preparations carried out at the licensed premises. It shall contain the following:-

1. General information

2. Personnel

3. Premises

4. Equipment

5. Sanitation

6. Documentation

7. Production

8. Quality control

9. Loan licence manufacture and licensee

10. Distribution, complaints and product recall

11. Self-Inspection

12. Export of drugs

7.4 PART IA

Specific Requirements For Manufacture of Sterile Products, Parenteral Preparations (Small Volume Injectables And Large Volume Parenterals) and Sterile Ophthalmic Preparations:

1. GENERAL

Sterile products, being very critical and sensitive in nature, a very high degree of precautions, prevention and preparations are needed.

Dampness, dirt and darkness are to be avoided to ensure aseptic conditions in all areas. There shall be strict compliance in the prescribed standards especially in the matter of supply of water, air, active materials and in the maintenance of hygienic environment.

2. BUILDINGS AND CIVIL WORKS

The Building shall be built on proper foundation with standardized materials to avoid cracks in critical areas like aseptic solution preparation, filling and sealing rooms. The manufacturing areas shall be clearly separated into support areas, preparation areas, change areas and aseptic areas.

In aseptic areas:

(a) Walls, floors and ceiling should be impervious, non-shedding, non flaking and non-cracking. Flooring should be unbroken and provided with a cove both at the junction between the wall and the floor as well as the wall and the ceiling

(b) Walls shall be flat, and ledges and recesses shall be avoided.

(c) Ceiling shall be solid and joints shall be sealed.

(d) Doors and Windows shall be made of non-shedding material(Aluminum or Steel material).

(e) The furniture used shall be smooth, washable and made of stainless steel.

The manufacturing and the support areas shall have the same quality of civil structure described above for aseptic areas, except the environmental standards which may vary in the critical areas.

Change rooms with entrance in the form of air-locks shall be provided before entry into the sterile product manufacturing areas and then to the aseptic area. Separate exit space from the aseptic areas is advisable.

3. AIR HANDLING SYSTEM (CENTRAL AIR-CONDITIONING)

Air handling units for sterile product manufacturing areas shall be different from those for other areas. Critical areas, such as the aseptic filing area, Sterilized components unloading area and change rooms conforming to Grades B, C and D respectively shall have separate air handling units. The filter configuration in the air handling system shall be suitably designed to achieve the grade of air as given in Table 1. Typical operational activities for clean areas are highlighted in Tables 2 and Table 3. The filling operations shall take place under Grade A conditions which shall be demonstrated under working of simulated conditions which shall be achieved by providing Laminar Air flow work stations with suitable HEPA filters or isolator technology.

TABLE 1: Air Borne Particulate Classification For Manufacture of Sterile Products

Grade	At rest		In operation	
	Maximum number of permitted particles per cubic meter equal to or above			
	0.5mm	5mm	0.5mm	5mm
A	3520	29	3500	29
B	35200	293	3.52,000	2930
C	352000	2930	3.52,0000	29300
D	3520000	29300	Not defined	Not defined

Table 2: Types of operations to be carried out in the various grades for aseptic preparation

Grade	Types of operation for aseptic preparations
A	Aseptic preparation and filling
B	Background room conditions for activities requiring Grade A
C	Preparation of solution to be filled
D	Handling of components after washing

Table 3 :Types of operation to be carried out in the various grades for terminally Sterilized products

Grade	Types of operations for terminally sterilized products
A	Filling of products, which are usually at risk.
C	Placement of filling and ceiling machines, preparation of solution, when usually at risk filling of product when unusually at risk.
D	Moulding, blowing (pre-forming) operations of plastic containers. Preparations of solutions and components for subsequent filling.

4. ENVIRONMENTAL MONITORING

All environmental parameters shall be verified and established at the time of installation and thereafter monitored at periodic intervals. There shall be a written environmental monitoring program and microbiological results shall be recorded, Recommended limits for microbiological monitoring of clean areas in operation are as given in the table 4.

Table 4 : Recommended Limits for Microbiological Monitoring of Clean Areas in Operation

Grade	Air sample cfu / m^3	Settle plate (dia.90mm. cfu/2hrs)	Contact plates (dia.55mm) cfu per plate	Glove points (five fingers) cfu per glove
A	< 1	< 1	< 1	< 1
B	10	5	5	5
C	100	50	25	-
D	500	100	50	-

5. GARMENTS

Outdoor clothing shall not be brought into the sterile areas. The garments shall be made of non-shedding and tight weave material cotton garments shall not be used. The garments shall shed virtually no fibers or particulate matter. Only clean, sterilized and protective garments shall be used at each work session. Gloves shall be made of latex or other suitable plastic in materials and shall be powder-free. The footwear shall be of suitable plastic or rubber material and shall be daily cleaned with a bactericide. Safety goggles or numbered glasses with side extensions shall be used inside aseptic areas. These shall be sanitized by a suitable method.

6. SANITATION

There shall be written procedures for the sanitation of sterile processing facilities. Employees carrying out sanitation of aseptic areas shall be trained specifically for this purpose. Different sanitizing agents shall be used in rotation and the concentrations of the same shall be as per the recommendations of the manufacturer. Records of rotational use of sanitizing agents shall be maintained. Cleaning of sterile processing facilities shall be undertaken with air suction devices or with non-linting sponges or clothes. Air particulate quality shall be evaluated on a regular basis and records maintained.

7. EQUIPMENT

Equipment for critical processes like aseptic filling and sterilizers shall be suitably validated according to a written program before putting them to use. Standard Operating Procedures shall be followed for each equipment for its calibration and operation and cleaning. Gauges and other measuring devices attached to equipment shall he calibrated at suitable intervals against a written program. The construction material used for the parts which are in direct contact with products and the manufacturing vessels may be stainless steel 316 or 316 mo-silicate glass (if glass containers) and the tubing shall be capable of being washed and autoclaved.

8. WATER AND STEAM SYSTEMS

Purified water shall he used for hand washing in change rooms. Containers, closures and machine parts may be washed with potable water followed by suitably filtered purified water.

Water for Injection for the manufacture of liquid injectables shall be freshly collected from the distillation plant or from a storage or circulation loop where the water, has been kept at above 70°C. Water for non-injectable sterile products like eye drops shall meet IP specifications for Purified water. Steam coming in contact with the product, primary containers and other product contact surfaces shall be sterile and pyrogen free.

9. MANUFACTURING PROCESS

Manufacture of sterile products shall be carried out only in areas under defined conditions. The time between the start of the preparation of the solution and its sterilization or filtration through a micro-organism retaining filter shall be minimized. Washed containers shall be sterilized immediately before use. Each lot of finished product shall be filled in one continuous operation. Special care shall be exercised while filling products in powder form so as not to contaminate the environment during transfer of powder to filling machine-hopper.

10. FORM -FILL -SEAL TECHNOLOGY OR BLOW- FILL-SEAL TECHNOLOGY

Form fill seal units are specially built automated machines in which through one continuous are formed from thermoplastic granules, filled and then sealed. Blow fill seal units are machines in which containers are moulded/blown (pre-formed) in separate clean rooms, by non-continuous operations. Preparation of primary packaging material such as glass bottles, ampoules and rubber stoppers shall be done in at least Grade D environment. Sterilization can be affected by moist or dry heat, by ethylene oxide (or other suitable gaseous Sterilizing agent), by filtration with subsequent aseptic filling in to sterile final containers, or by irradiation with ionizing radiation.

11. PRODUCT CONTAINERS AND CLOSURES

All containers and closures intended for use shall comply with the pharmacopoeial and other specified requirements. All containers and closures shall be rinsed prior to sterilization with water for injection according to written procedure. The design of closures, containers and stoppers shall be such as to make cleaning, easy and also to make an airtight seal when fitted to the bottles. Glass bottles made of USP Type-I and USP Type-II glass shall only be used. Pre-formed plastic containers intended to be used for the packing of Large Volume Parenteral shall be moulded in-house by one continuous operation through an automatic machine. The rubber stoppers used for Large Volume Parenterals shall comply with specifications prescribed in the current edition of the Indian Pharmacopoeia.

12. DOCUMENTATION

Products shall be released only after complete filling and testing. Result of the tests relating to sterility, pyrogens and Bacterial endotoxins shall be maintained in the analytical records. Validation details and simulation trial records shall be maintained separately. Records of environmental monitoring like temperature, humidity, microbiological data etc, shall be maintained. Records of periodic servicing of HEPA filters, sterilizers and other periodic maintenance of facilities and equipment carried out shall also be maintained.

7.5 PART 1B

SPECIFIC REQUIREMENTS FOR MANUFACTURE OF ORAL SOLID DOSAGE FORMS (TABLETS AND CAPSULES)

1. GENERAL

The processing of dry materials and products creates problems of dust control and cross-contamination. Special attention is, therefore, needed in the design, maintenance and use of premises and equipment in order to overcome these problems. Suitable environmental conditions for the products handled shall be maintained by installation of air-conditioning wherever necessary. Effective air-extraction systems, with discharge points situated to avoid contamination of other products and processes shall be provided. Filters shall be installed to retain dust and to protect the factory and local environment. Where the facilities are designed to provide special environmental conditions of pressure differentials between rooms, these conditions shall be regularly monitored and any specification results brought to the immediate attention of the production and quality assurance departments which shall be immediately attended to care shall be taken to guard against any material lodging and remaining undetected in any processing or packaging equipment. Particular care shall be taken to ensure that any vacuum, compressed air or an extraction nozzle are kept clean and that there is no evidence of lubricants leaking into the product from any part of the equipments.

2. SIFTING, MIXING AND GRANULATION

Unless operated as a closed system mixing, sifting and blending equipments shall be fitted with dust extractors. Residues from sieving operations shall be examined periodically for evidence of the presence of unwanted materials. Critical operating parameters like time and temperature for each mixing blending and drying operation shall be specified in a Master Formula monitored during processing, and recorded in the batch records. Air entering the drier shall be filtered. Granulation and coating solutions shall be made, stored and used in a manner which minimizes the risk of contamination or microbial growth.

3. COMPRESSION (TABLETS)

Each tablet compressing machine shall be provided with effective dust control facilities to avoid cross contamination. Suitable physical, procedural and labeling arrangements shall be made to prevent mix-up of materials, granules and tablets on compression machinery. Accurate and calibrated weighing equipment shall be readily available and used for in-process monitoring of tablet weight variation. At the commencement of each compression run and in case of multiple compression points in a compression machine, sufficient individual tablets shall be examined at fixed intervals to ensure that a tablet from each compression station or from each compression point has been inspected for suitable pharmacopoeial parameters like 'appearance', weight variation', 'disintegration', 'hardness', 'friability' and 'thickness'. The results shall be recorded as part of the batch documentation.

4. COATING (TABLETS)

Air supplied to coating pans for doing purposes shall be filtered air and or suitable quality. The area shall be provided with suitable exhaust system and environmental control (temperature. humidity) measures. Coating solutions and suspensions shall be made afresh and used in a manner, which shall minimize the risk of microbial growth. Their preparation and use shall be documented and recorded.

5. FILLING OF HARD GELATIN CAPSULE

Empty capsules shells shall be regarded as 'drug component' and treated accordingly. They shall be stored under conditions which shall ensure their safety from the effects of excessive heat and moisture.

6. PRINTING (TABLETS AND CAPSULES)

Special care shall he taken to avoid product mix-up during any printing of tablets and capsules. Where different products or different batches of the same product are printed simultaneously, the operations shall adequately be segregated. Edible grade colours and suitable printing ink shall be used for such printing. After printing, tablets and capsules shall be approved by quality control before release for packaging or sale.

7. PACKAGING (STRIP AND BLISTER)

Care. shall be taken when using automatic tablet and capsule counting, strip and blister packaging equipment to ensure that all 'rogue' tablets capsules or foils from packaging operation are removed before a new packaging operation is commenced. There shall be an independent recorded check of the equipment before a new batch of tablets or capsules is handled. The strips coming out of the machine shall be inspected for defects such as misprint, cuts on the foil, missing tablets and improper sealing. Integrity of individual packaging strips and blisters shall be subjected to vacuum test periodically to ensure leak proofness of each pocket strip and blister and records maintained.

7.6 PART IC

SPECIFIC REQUIREMENTS FOR MANUFACTURE OF ORAL LIQUIDS (SYRUPS, ELIXIRS, EMULSIONS AND SUSPENSIONS)

1. BUILDING AND EQUIPMENT

The premises and equipment shall be designed, constructed and maintained to suit the manufacturing of Oral Liquids. The layout and design of the manufacturing area shall strive to minimize the risk of cross contamination and mix-ups. Manufacturing area shall have entry through double door air-lock facility. It shall be made fly proof by use of 'fly catcher' and/or 'air curtain'. Tanks, containers, pipe work and pumps shall be designed and installed so that they can be easily cleaned and sanitized. Equipment design shall be such as to prevent accumulation of residual microbial growth or cross-contamination. Stainless Steel or any other appropriate material shall be used for parts of equipments coming in direct contact with the products. Arrangements for cleaning of containers, closures and droppers shall be made with the help of suitable machines/devices equipped with high pressure air, water and steam jets.

2. PURIFIED WATER

The chemical and microbiological quality of purified water used shall be specified and monitored routinely. There shall be a written procedure for operation and maintenance of the purified water system. Care shall he taken to avoid the risk of microbial proliferation with appropriate methods like recirculation, use of UV treatment, treatment with heat and sanitizing agent. After any chemical sanitization of the water system, a flushing shall be done to ensure that the Sanitizing agent has been effectively removed.

3. MANUFACTURING

Manufacturing personnel shall wear non-fiber shedding clothing to prevent contamination of the product. Care shall be taken to maintain the homogeneity of emulsion by use of appropriate emulsifier and suspensions by use of appropriate stirrer during filling. Mixing and tilling processes shall be specified and monitored. Special care shall be taken at the beginning of the filling process, after stoppage due to any interruption and at the end of the process to ensure that the product is uniformly homogenous during the filling process. The primary packaging area shall have an air supply which is filtered through 5 micron filters. The temperature of the area shall not exceed 30°C. When the bulk product is not immediately packed, the maximum period of storage and storage conditions shall be as specified in the master formula. The maximum period of storage time of a product in the bulk stage shall be validated.

7.7 PART ID

SPECIFIC REQUIREMENTS FOR MANUFACTURE OF TOPICAL PRODUCTS i.e. EXTERNAL PREPARATIONS (CREAMS, OINTMENTS, PASTES, EMULSIONS,LOTIONS, SOLUTIONS, DUSTING POWDERS AND IDENTICAL PRODUCTS)

1. The entrance to the area where topical products are manufactured shall be through a suitable airlock. Outside the airlock, insectocutors shall be installed.

2. The air to this manufacturing area shall be filtered through at least 20 air filters and shall be air-conditioned. The area shall be ventilated.

3. The area shall be fitted with an exhaust system of suitable capacity to effectively remove vapours. fumes, smoke, floating dust particles.

4. The equipment used shall be designed and maintained to prevent the product from being accidentally contaminated with any foreign matter or lubricant.

5. No rags or dusters shall be used in the process of cleaning or drying the process equipment or accessories used.

6. Water used in compounding shall be Purified Water IP.

7. Powders, whenever used, shall be suitably sieved before use.

8. Heating vehicles and a base like petroleum jelly shall be done in separate mixing area in suitable stainless steel vessels, using steam, gas, electricity, solar energy etc.

9. A Separate packing section may be provided for primary packaging of the products.

7.8 PART 1E

SPECIFIC REQUIREMENTS FOR MANUFACTURE OF METERED-DOSE INHALERS (MDI)

1. GENERAL

Manufacture of Metered-Dose Inhalers shall be done under conditions which shall ensure minimum microbial and particulate contamination. Assurance of the quality of components and bulk product is very important. Where medicaments are in suspended state, uniformity of suspension shall be established.

2. BUILDING AND CIVIL WORKS

The building shall be located on a solid foundation to reduce risk of cracking walls and floor due to the movement of equipment and machinery. All building surfaces shall he impervious, smooth and non shedding. Flooring shall be continuous and provided with a cove between the floor and the wall as well the wall to the ceiling. Ceiling shall be solid, continuous and covered to walls. The manufacturing area shall be segregated into change rooms for personnel, container preparation area, bulk preparations and filling area, quarantine area and spray testing and packing areas. The propellants used for manufacture shall be delivered to the manufacturing area distribution system by filtering them through 2μ filters. The bulk containers of propellants shall be stored, suitably identified, away from the manufacturing facilities.

3. ENVIRONMENTAL CONDITIONS

The requirements of temperature and humidity in the manufacturing area shall be decided depending on the type of product and propellants handled in the facility. There shall be a difference in room pressure between the manufacturing area and the support areas and the differential pressure shall be not less than 15 Pascals, (0.06 inches or 1.5 mm Water gauge). There shall be a written schedule for the monitoring of environmental conditions. Temperature and humidity shall be monitored daily.

4. GARMENTS

Personnel in the manufacturing and filling section shall wear suitable single-piece-garment made out of non-shedding tight weave material. Personnel in support areas shall wear clean factory uniforms. Gloves made of suitable material having no interaction with the propellants shall be used by the operators in the manufacturing and filing areas. Suitable department-specific personnel protective equipment like footwear and safety glasses shall be used wherever hazard exists.

5. SANITATION

There shall be written procedures for the sanitation of the MDI manufacturing facility. Special care should be taken to handle residues and rinses of propellants. Use of water for cleaning shall be restricted and controlled. Routinely used disinfectants are suitable for sanitizing the different areas. Records of sanitation shall be maintained.

6. EQUIPMENT

Manufacturing equipment shall be closed system. The vessels and supply lines shall he stainless steel. Suitable check weights, spray testing machines and labeling machines shall be provided in the department. All the equipment shall be suitably calibrated and their performance validated on receipt and thereafter periodically.

7. MANUFACTURE

There shall be an approved Master Formula Records for the manufacture of metered dose inhalers. All propellants, liquids and gasses shall be filtered through 2 p. filters to remove particles. The primary packing material shall be appropriately cleaned by compressed air suitably filtered through 0.2 µ filter. The humidity of the compressed air shall be controlled as applicable. The valves shall he carefully handled and after de-cartooning, these shall be kept in clean, closed containers in the filing room. For suspensions, the bulk shall be kept stirred continuously. In-process controls shall include periodical checking of weight of bulk formulation filed in the containers. In a two-shot-filling process (liquid filling followed by gaseous filling), it shall be ensured that 100% check on weight is carried out. Filled containers shall be quarantined for a suitable period established by the manufacturer to detect leaking containers prior to testing, labelling and packing.

8. DOCUMENTATION

In addition to the routine good manufacturing practices documentation, manufacturing records shall show the following additional information:

(1) Temperature and humidity in the manufacturing area.

(2) Periodic filled weights of the formulation.

(3) Records of rejections during on line check weighing.

(4) Records of rejection during spray testing.

7.9 PART IF

SPECIFIC REQUIREMENTS OF PREMISES, PLANT AND MATERIALS FOR MANUFACTURE OF ACTIVE PHARMACEUTICAL INGREDIENTS (BULK DRUGS)

1. BUILDINGS AND CIVIL WORKS

The final stage of preparation of a drug, like isolation/filtration/drying/milling/sieving and packing operations shall be provided with air filtration systems including pre-filters and finally with a 5 micron filter. Air handling systems with adequate number of air changes per hour or any other suitable system to control the air borne contamination shall be provided. Humidity/Temperature shall also be controlled for all the operations wherever required. Ancillary area shall be provided for boiler-house. Utility areas like heat exchangers, chilling workshop, store and supply of gases shall also be provided. The requirements for the sterile active pharmaceutical ingredient shall be in line with the facilities required for formulations to be filled aseptically.

2. STERILE PRODUCTS

Sterile active pharmaceutical ingredient filled aseptically shall be treated as formulation from the stage wherever the process demands like crystallisation, Iyophilisation, filtration etc. All conditions applicable to formulations that are required to be filled aseptically shall be applicable for the manufacture of sterile active pharmaceutical ingredients.

3. UTILITIES/SERVICES

Equipment like chilling plant, boiler, heat exchangers, vacuum and gas storage vessels shall be serviced. Cleaned, sanitized and maintained at appropriate intervals to prevent malfunctions or contamination that may interfere with safety, identity, strength, quality or purity of the drug product.

4. EQUIPMENT DESIGN, SIZE AND LOCATION

Equipment used in the manufacture, processing, packing or holding of an active pharmaceutical ingredient shall be of appropriate design, adequate size and suitably located to facilitate operations for its intended use and for its cleaning and maintenance. A written procedures shall be established and followed for cleaning and maintenance of equipment, including utensils used in the manufacture, processing, packing or holding of active pharmaceutical ingredients.

5. IN-PROCESS CONTROLS

In-process controls for chemical reactions and In-process controls for physical operations are tested for quality attributes and approved or rejected by the quality control unit.

6. PRODUCT CONTAINERS AND CLOSURES

All containers and closures intended for use shall comply with the pharmacopoeial and other specified requirements. Container closure system shall provide adequate protection against foreseeable external factors in storage/transportation and use that may cause deterioration or contamination of the active pharmaceutical ingredient. Bulk containers and closures shall be cleaned and, where indicated by the nature of the active pharmaceutical ingredient, sterilized to ensure that they are suitable for their intended use.

7.10 PART II

REQUIREMENTS OF PLANT AND EQUIPMENT

1. EXTERNAL PREPARATIONS

The following equipment is recommended for the manufacture of external preparations i.e., ointments, emulsion, lotions, solutions, pastes, creams, dusting powders and such identical products used for external applications whichever is applicable, namely:

Mixing and storage tanks (Stainless steel), Jacketed Kettle (steam, gas or electrically heated),

Mixer (Electrically operated), Planetary mixer, A colloid mill or a suitable emulsifier, A triple roller mill or an ointment mill, Liquid filling equipment (Electrically operated), Jar on table filling equipment (Electrically operated).

Area:— (1) A minimum area of thirty square meters for basic installation and ten square meters for Ancillary area is recommended.

(2) Areas for formulations meant for external use and internal use shall be separately proved to avoid mix up.

2. ORAL LIQUID PREPARATIONS

The following equipment is recommended for the manufacture of oral/internal use preparations, i.e., syrups, elixirs, emulsions and suspensions whichever is applicable namely:

Mixing and storage tanks (Stainless steel), Jacketted Kettle/ Stainless steel tanks (steam, gas or electrically heated), Portable stirrer (Electrically operated), A colloid mill or a suitable emulsifier (Electrically operated), Suitable filtration equipment (Electrically operated), Semi automatic/automatic bottle filling machine, Pilfer proof cap sealing machine, Water distillation unit. or deionizer, Clarity testing inspection units.

Area:— A minimum area of thirty square meters for basic installation and ten square meters for ancillary area is recommended.

3. TABLETS

The tableting section shall be free from dust and floating particles and may be air conditioned. For this purpose each tablet machine shall be isolated into cubicles and connected to a vacuum dust collector or an exhaust system for effective operations, the tablet production department shall be divided into four distinct and separate sections as follows:—

(a) Mixing, Granulation and Drying section.

(b) Tablet compression section.

(c) Packaging section (strip/blister machine wherever required).

(d) Coating section (wherever required).

The following electrically operated equipment are recommended for the manufacture of compressed tablets and hypodermic tablets. in each of the above sectiohs, namely:

(a) **Granulation-cum-Drying section:** Disintegrator and sifter, Power mixer, Mass mixer/ Planetery mixer/Rapid mixer granulator, Granulator, Thermostatically controlled hot air oven with trays(preferably mounted on a trolley)/Fluid bed dryer, Weighing machines.

(b) **Compression section:** Tablet compression machine (single/ multi punch/ rotatory), Punch and dies storage cabinets, Tablet de-duster, Tablet inspection unit/belt, Dissolution test apparatus, In-process testing equipment like single pan electronic balance, hardness tester, friability and disintegration test apparatus, Air-conditioning and dehumidification arrangement.

(c) **Packaging section:** Strip/blister packaging machine, Leak test apparatus (vacuum system), Tablet counters, Air-conditioning and dehumidification arrangement.

Area:— A minimum area of sixty square meters for basic installation and twenty square meters for Ancillary area is recommended for an coated tablets.

(d) **Coating section:** Jacketed kettle (steam, gas, or electrically heated for preparing coating suspension), Coating pan (Stainless steel),

Polishing pan , Exhaust system (including vacuum dust collector), Air-conditioning and Dehumidification Arrangement, Weighing balance.

The coating section shall be made dust free with suitable exhaust system to remove excess powder and fumes resulting from solvent evaporation it shall be air-conditioned and dehumidified wherever considered necessary.

Area:—A minimum additional area of thirty square metres for coating section for basic installation and ten square meters for ancillary area is recommended.

4. POWDERS

The following equipment is recommended for the manufacture of powders namely:

Disintegrator, Mixer, Sifter, Stainless steel vessels and scoops of suitable sizes, Filling equipment, Weighing balance.

Area:—A minimum area of thirty square metres is recommended to allow for the basic installations. Where the actual blending is to be done on the premises, an additional room shall be provided for the purpose.

5. CAPSULES

For the manufacture of capsules separate enclosed area suitably air-conditioned and dehumidified with an airlock arrangement shall be provided. The following equipment is recommended for filling Hard Gelatin Capsules namely:

Mixing and blending equipment , Capsule filling units, Capsules counters, Weighing balance, Disintegration test apparatus, Capsule polishing equipment,

Area:—A minimum area of twenty five square metres for basic installation and ten square metres for Ancillary area each for penicillin and non-penicillin sections is recommended.

6. SURGICAL DRESSING

The following equipment is recommended for the manufacture of surgical dressings other than Absorbent Cotton Wool, namely:

Rolling machine, Trimming machine,Cutting equipment, Folding and pressing machine for gauze,Mixing tanks for processing medicated dressing, Hot air dry oven, Steam sterilizer or dry heat sterilizer or other suitable equipment,Work tablets/benches for different operations.

Area:—A minimum area of thirty square meters is recommended to allow for the basic installations. In case medicated dressings are to be manufactured, another room with a minimum area of thirty square shall be provided.

7. OPHTHALMIC PREPARATIONS

For the manufacture of Ophthalmic preparations separate enclosed areas with air lock arrangement shall be provided. The following equipment is recommended for manufacture under aseptic conditions of Eye-Ointments, Eye lotions and other preparations for external use, namely:

Thermostatically controlled hot air ovens , Jacketted kettle/ Stainless steel tanks , Mixing and storage tanks of stainless steel/Planetry mixer, Colloid mill or ointment mill, Tube filling and crimping equipment (semi-automatic or automatic filling machines), Tube cleaning equipment (air jet type), Tube washing and drying equipment, Automatic vial washing machine, Vial drying oven, Rubber bung washing machine, Sintered glass funnel, seitz or filter candle ,Liquid filling equipment , Autoclave , Air-conditioning and dehumidification arrangement , Laminar air flow units.

Area:—(1) A minimum area of twenty five square meters for basic installations and ten square meters for Ancillary area is recommended.

8. PESSARIES AND SUPPOSITORIES

The following equipment is recommended for manufacture of Pessaries and Suppositories. namely:-

Mixing and pouring equipment, Moulding equipment, Weighing devices.

Area:—A minimum area of twenty square meters is recommended to allow for the basic installation.

9. INHALERS AND VITRALLAE

The following equipment is recommended for manufacture of inhalers and vitrallae, namely:

Mixing equipment, Graduated delivery equipment for measurement of the medicament during filling. Sealing equipment.

Area:—An area of minimum twenty square metres is recommended for the basic installations.

10. REPACKING OF DRUGS AND PHARMACEUTICAL CHEMICALS

The following equipment is recommended for repacking of drugs and pharmaceuticals, chemicals. namely:

Powder disintegrator, Powder sifter, Stainless steel scoops and vessels of suitable sizes, Weighing and measuring equipment, Filling equipment (semi-automatic/automatic machine), Electric sealing machine.

Area:—An area of minimum of thirty square meters is recommended for the basic installation. In case of operations involving floating particles of fine powder, a suitable exhaust system shall be provided.

11.PARENTERAL PREPARATIONS:

11.1.Parenteral preparations in glass containers:

The following equipment is recommended for Parenteral preparations in glass containers, namely:

(a) **Water management area:** De-ionised water treatment unit, Distillation unit, Thermostatically controlled water storage tank, Transfer pumps, Stainless steel service lines for carrying water into user areas.

(b) Containers and closures preparation area: Automatic rotary ampoule/vial/bottle washing machine having separate air, water, distilled water jets, Automatic closures washing machine, Storage equipment for ampoules. vials, bottles and closures, Dryer/sterilizer, dust proof storage cabinets, Stainless steel benches/stools.

(c) Solution preparation area: Solution preparation and mixing Stainless steel tanks and other containers, Portable–stirrer, Filtration equipment with cartridge and membrane, filters/bacteriological filters, Transfer pumps, Stainless steel benches/stools.

(d) Filling. capping and sealing area: Automatic ampoule/vial/bottle filling, sealing and capping machine under laminar air flow work station, Gas lines, Stainless steel benches/stools.

(e) Sterilization area: Steam sterilizer, Hot Air sterilizer , Pressure leak test apparatus.

(f) Quarantine area: Storage cabinets, Raised platforms/steel racks.

(g) Visual inspection area:Visual inspection units , Stainless steel benches/stools.

(h) Packaging area: Batch coding machine,Labeling unit ,benches/ stools.

Area:—(1)A minimum area of one hundred and fifty square meters for the basic installation and an ancillary area of one hundred square metres for small volume injectables is recommended. For large volume parenterals an area of one hundred and fifty square metres each for the basic installation and for ancillary area is recommended.

(2) Areas for formulations meant for external use and internal use shall be separately provided to avoid mix up.

(3) Packaging materials for large volume parenteral shall have a minimum area of 100 square metres.

11.2 Parenteral preparations in Plastic containers by Form-Fill-Seal/Blow, Fill-Seal technology

The following equipment is recommended for Parenteral preparations in in Plastic containers, namely:

(a) Water management area: De-ionised water treatment unit, Distillation unit, Thermostatically controlled water storage tank,Transfer pumps, Stainless steel service lines for carrying water into user areas.

(b) Solution preparation area: Storage tanks, Transfer pumps, Cartridge and membrane filters.

(c) Container moulding-cum-filling and sealing area: Sterile Form-Fill-Seal machine, Feeding-cum-filling tank.

(d) Sterilization area: Super heated steam sterilizer .

(e) Quarantine area: Adequate number of platforms/racks with storage system.

(f) Visual inspection area : Visual inspection unit.

(g) Packaging area: Pressure leak test apparatus , Batch coding machine, Labelling unit.

Area:—(1) A minimum area of two hundred and fifty square metres for the basic installation and an Ancillary area of one hundred and fifty square metres for large volume parenteral preparations in plastic containers by Form-Fill-Seal technology is recommended.

(2) Areas for formulations meant for external use and internal use shall be separately provided to avoid mix up.

(3) Packaging materials for large volume parenteral shall have a minimum area of 100 square meters.

7.11 USFDA GMP

US FDA introduced certain Practices to regulate the manufacturing and testing of pharmaceutical products aiming at their quality and safety in the form of GMPs in 1963. Although it took about eight years (1971) to revise them, they are in no way stagnant. Regulation defined the "GMP as a system for ensuring that products are consistently produced and controlled according to quality standards. It is designed to minimize the risks involved in any pharmaceutical production that cannot be eliminated through testing the final product". Owing to the dynamic nature of the GMPs, In the year 1976, the term cGMP came into existence. The law recognizes that Current Good manufacturing practice (cGMP) with the attendant Quality control procedures are paramount to the production of quality products. The next revision of the cGMP took palace in 1978, and these are in effect at present. In fact, the word "Current" in referring to suggest that they are dynamic and the regulatory agency constantly updates and maintains them in relation to the current state of the art and science of drug manufacturing practice in the revision. cGMP is defined as a requirement that drugs, and the methods used in, or the facilities or controls used in their manufacturer, processing, packing or holding conform with those practice that will assure that such drugs meet the requirement of the act as to safety, and have the identity, strength, quality, and purity characteristics.

The current regulations are covered in Code of Federal Regulations (CFR).

7.12 CODE OF FEDERAL REGULATIONS (CFR)

The Code of Federal Regulations (CFR) is a codification of the general and permanent rules of the federal government. The CFR contains the complete and official text of the regulations that are enforced by federal agencies. The CFR is divided into 50 titles that represent broad areas subject to the Federal regulations. Each title is divided into chapters that are assigned to various agencies issuing regulations pertaining to that broad subject area. Each chapter is divided into parts covering specific regulatory areas. Each part or subpart is then divided into sections, the basic unit of the CFR. Citations pertaining to specific information in the CFR will usually be provided at the section level. Each volume of the CFR is updated once each calendar year and is issued on a quarterly basis. Parts 210 & 211 are updated each April.

The CFR's that relate to cGMP in the pharmaceutical and biotechnology companies are:

- 21 CFR Part 210 - Current Good Manufacturing Practice in Manufacturing, Processing, Packing, or Holding of Drugs.

- 21 CFR Part 211 - Current Good Manufacturing Practice for Finished Pharmaceuticals.

7.13 TITLE 21—FOOD AND DRUGS

CHAPTER I—FOOD AND DRUG ADMINISTRATION DEPARTMENT OF HEALTH AND HUMAN SERVICES

SUBCHAPTER C—DRUGS: GENERAL

PART 210—CURRENT GOOD MANUFACTURING PRACTICE IN MANUFACTURING, PROCESSING, PACKING, OR HOLDING OF DRUGS; GENERAL

Part 210 is divided into three sections

210.1 Status of current good manufacturing practice regulations.

210.2 Applicability of current good manufacturing practice regulations.

210.3 Definitions

210.1 Status of current good manufacturing practice regulations

(a)The regulations set forth in this part and in parts 211 through 226 of this chapter contain the minimum current good manufacturing practice for methods to be used in, and the facilities or controls to be used for, the manufacture, processing, packing, or holding of a drug to assure that such drug meets the requirements of the act as to safety, and has the identity and strength and meets the quality and purity characteristics that it purports or is represented to possess.

(b)The failure to comply with any regulation set forth in this part and in parts 211 through 226 of this chapter in the manufacture, processing, packing, or holding of a drug shall render such drug to be adulterated under section 501(a)(2)(B) of the act and such drug, as well as the person who is responsible for the failure to comply, shall be subject to regulatory action.

(c) Owners and operators of establishments engaged in the recovery, donor screening, testing (including donor testing), processing, storage, labeling, packaging, or distribution of human cells, tissues, and cellular and tissue based products (HCT/Ps), as defined in § 1271.3(d) of this chapter, that are drugs (subject to review under an application submitted under section 505 of the act or under a biological product license application under section 351 of the Public Health Service Act), are subject to the donor-eligibility and applicable current good tissue practice procedures set forth in part 1271 subparts C and D of this chapter, in addition to the regulations in this part and in parts 211 through 226 of this chapter. Failure to comply with any applicable regulation set forth in this part, in parts 211 through 226 of this chapter, inpart 1271 subpart C of this chapter, or in part 1271 subpart D of this chapter with respect to the manufacture, processing, packing or holding of a drug, renders an HCT/P adulterated under section 501(a)(2)(B) of the act. Such HCT/P, as well as the person who is responsible for the failure to comply, is subject to regulatory action.

210.2 Applicability of current good manufacturing practice regulations

(a)The regulations in this part and in parts 211 through 226 of this chapter as they may pertain to a drug; in parts 600 through 680 of this chapter as they may pertain to a biological product for human use; and in part 1271 of this chapter as they are applicable to a human cell, tissue, or cellular or tissue based product that is a drug shall be considered to supplement, not supersede, each other, unless the regulations explicitly provide otherwise. In the event of a conflict between applicable regulations in this part and in other parts of this chapter, the regulation specifically applicable to the drug product in question shall supersede the more general.

(b) If a person engages in only some operations subject to the regulations in this part, in parts 211 through 226 of this chapter, in parts 600 through 680 of this chapter, and in part 1271 of this chapter, and not in others, that person need only comply with those regulations applicable to the operations in which he or she is engaged.

(c)An investigational drug for use in a phase 1 study, as described in § 312.21(a) of this chapter, is subject tothe statutory requirements set forth in 21 U.S.C. 351(a)(2)(B). The production of such drug is exempt from compliance with the regulations in part 211 of this chapter. However, this exemption does not apply to an investigational drug for use in a phase 1 study once the investigational drug has been made available for use by or for the sponsor in a phase 2 or phase 3 study, as described in § 312.21(b) and (c) of this chapter, or the drug has been lawfully marketed. If the investigational drug has been made available in a phase 2 or phase 3 study or the drug has been lawfully marketed, the drug for use in the phase 1 study must comply with part 211.

210.3 Definitions

(a) The definitions and interpretations contained in section 201 of the act shall be applicable to such terms when used in this part and in parts 211 through 226 of this chapter.

(b) The following definitions of terms apply to this part and to parts 211through 226 of this chapter.

(1) **Act** means the Federal Food, Drug,and Cosmetic Act, as amended (21U.S.C. 301 et seq.).

(2) **Batch** means a specific quantity of a drug or other material that is intended to have uniform character and quality, within specified limits, and is produced according to a single manufacturing order during the same cycle of manufacture.

(3) **Component** means any ingredient intended for use in the manufacture of a drug product, including those that may not appear in such drug product.

(4) **Drug product** means a finished dosage form, for example, tablet, capsule, solution, etc., that contains an active drug ingredient generally, but not necessarily,in association with inactive ingredients. The term also includes a finished dosage form that does not contain an active ingredient but is intended to be used as a placebo.

(5) **Fiber** means any particulate contaminant with a length at least three times greater than its width.

(6) **Nonfiber releasing filter** means any filter, which after appropriate pretreatment such as washing or flushing, will not release fibers

into the component or drug product that is being filtered.

(7) **Active ingredient** means any component that is intended to furnish pharmacological activity or other direct effect in the diagnosis, cure, mitigation, treatment, or prevention of disease, or to affect the structure or any function of the body of man or other animals. The term includes those components that may undergo chemical change in the manufacture of the drug product and be present in the drug product in a modified form intended to furnish the specified activity or effect.

(8) **Inactive ingredient** means any component other than an active ingredient.

(9) **In-process material** means any material fabricated, compounded, blended, or derived by chemical reaction that is produced for, and used in, the preparation of the drug product.

(10) **Lot** means a batch, or a specific identified portion of a batch, having uniform character and quality within specified limits; or, in the case of a drug product produced by continuous process, it is a specific identified amount produced in a unit of time or quantity in a manner that assures its having uniform character and quality within specified limits.

(11) **Lot number, control number, or batch number** means any distinctive combination of letters, numbers, or symbols, or any combination of them, from which the complete history of the manufacture, processing, packing, holding, and distribution of a batch or lot of drug product or other material can be determined.

(12) **Manufacture, processing, packing, or holding of a drug product** includes packaging and labeling operations, testing, and quality control of drug products.

(13) The term **medicated feed** means any Type B or Type C medicated feed as defined in § 558.3 of this chapter. The feed contains one or more drugs as defined in section 201(g) of the act. The manufacture of medicated feeds is subject to the requirements of part 225 of this chapter.

(14) The term **medicated premix** means a Type A medicated article as defined in § 558.3 of this chapter. The article contains one or more drugs as defined in section 201(g) of the act. The manufacture of medicated premixes is subject to the requirements of part 226 of this chapter.

(15) **Quality control unit** means any person or organizational element designated by the firm to be responsible for the duties relating to quality control.

(16) **Strength means**: (i) The concentration of the drug substance (for example, weight/weight, weight/volume, or unit dose/volume basis), and/or (ii) The potency, that is, the therapeutic activity of the drug product as indicated by appropriate laboratory tests or by adequately developed and controlled clinical data (expressed, for example, in terms of units by reference to a standard).

(17) **Theoretical yield** means the quantity that would be produced at any appropriate phase of manufacture, process sing, or packing of a particular drug product, based upon the quantity of components to be used, in the absence of any loss or error in actual production.

(18) **Actual yield** means the quantity that is actually produced at any appropriate phase of manufacture, processing, or packing of a particular drug product.

(19) **Percentage of theoretical yield** means the ratio of the actual yield (at any appropriate phase of manufacture, processing, or packing of a particular drug product) to the theoretical yield(at the same phase), stated as a percentage.

(20) **Acceptance criteria** means the product specifications and acceptance/rejection criteria, such as acceptable quality level and unacceptable quality level, with an associated sampling plan, that are necessary for making a decision to accept or reject a lot or batch (or any other convenient subgroups of manufactured units).

(21) **Representative sample** means a sample that consists of a number of units that are drawn based on rational criteria such as

random sampling and intended to assure that the sample accurately portrays the material being sampled.

(22) **Gang-printed labeling** means labeling derived from a sheet of material on which more than one item of labeling is printed.

PART 211—CURRENT GOOD MANUFACTURING PRACTICE FOR FINISHED PHARMACEUTICALS

Part 211 is divided into 11 sub parts. Each subpart is again divided into sections.

Subpart A—General Provisions

211.1 - Scope.

211.3 - Definitions.

Subpart B—Organization and Personnel

211.22 - Responsibilities of quality control unit.

211.25 - Personnel qualifications.

211.28 - Personnel responsibilities.

211.34 - Consultants.

Subpart C—Buildings and Facilities

211.42 - Design and construction features.

211.44 - Lighting.

211.46 - Ventilation, air filtration, air heating and cooling.

211.48 - Plumbing.

211.50 - Sewage and refuse.

211.52 - Washing and toilet facilities.

211.56 - Sanitation.

211.58 - Maintenance.

Subpart D—Equipment

211.63 - Equipment design, size, and location.

211.65 - Equipment construction.

211.67 - Equipment cleaning and maintenance.

211.68 - Automatic, mechanical, and electronic equipment.

211.72 - Filters.

Subpart E—Control of Components and Drug Product Containers and Closures

211.80 - General requirements.

211.82 - Receipt and storage of untested components, drug product containers, and closures.

211.84 - Testing and approval or rejection of components, drug product containers, and closures.

211.86 - Use of approved components, drug product containers, and closures.

211.87 - Retesting of approved components, drug product containers, and closures.

211.89 - Rejected components, drug product containers, and closures.

211.94 - Drug product containers and closures.

Subpart F—Production and Process Controls

211.100 - Written procedures; deviations.

211.101 - Charge-in of components.

211.103 - Calculation of yield.

211.105 - Equipment identification.

211.110 - Sampling and testing of in-process materials and drug products.

Subpart K—Returned and Salvaged Drug Products

Subpart A—General Provisions

211.1 – Scope

The regulations in this part contain the minimum current good manufacturing practice for preparation of drug products for administration to humans or animals.

211.3 – **Definitions:** The definitions set forth in 210.3 of this chapter apply in this part.

Subpart B—Organization and Personnel

211.22 - Responsibilities of quality control unit

(a) There shall be a quality control unit that shall have the responsibility and authority to approve or reject all components, drug product containers, closures, in-process materials, packaging material, labeling, and drug products, and the authority to review production records to assure that no errors have occurred or, if errors have occurred, that they have been fully investigated. The quality control unit shall be responsible for approving or rejecting drug products manufactured, processed, packed, or held under contract by another company.

(b) Adequate laboratory facilities for the testing and approval (or rejection) of components, drug product containers, closures, packaging materials, in-process materials, and drug products shall be available to the quality control unit.

(c) The quality control unit shall have the responsibility for approving or rejecting all procedures or specifications impacting on the identity, strength, quality, and purity of the drug product.

(d) The responsibilities and procedures applicable to the quality control unit shall be in writing; such written procedures shall be followed.

211.25 Personnel qualifications

(a) Each person engaged in the manufacture, processing, packing, or holding of a drug product shall have education, training, and experience, or any combination thereof, to enable that person to perform the assigned functions. Training shall be in the particular operations that the employee performs and in current good manufacturing practice (including the current good manufacturing practice regulations in this chapter and written procedures required by these regulations) as they relate to the employee's functions. Training in current good manufacturing practice shall be conducted by qualified individuals on a continuing basis and with sufficient frequency to assure that employees remain familiar with cGMP requirements applicable to them.

(b) Each person responsible for supervising the manufacture, processing, packing, or holding of a drug product shall have the education, training, and experience, or any combination thereof, to perform assigned functions in such a manner as to provide assurance that the drug product has the safety, identity, strength, quality, and purity that it purports or is represented to possess.

(c) There shall be an adequate number of qualified personnel to perform and supervise the manufacture, processing, packing, or holding of each drug product.

211.28 Personnel responsibilities

(a) Personnel engaged in the manufacture, processing, packing, or holding of a drug product shall wear clean clothing appropriate for the duties they perform. Protective apparel, such as head, face, hand, and arm coverings,shall be worn as necessary to protect drug products from contamination.

(b) Personnel shall practice good sanitation and health habits.

(c) Only personnel authorized by supervisory personnel shall enter those areas of the buildings and facilities designated as limited-access areas.

(d) Any person shown at any time (either by medical examination or supervisory observation) to have an apparent illness or open lesions that may adversely affect the safety or quality of drug products shall be excluded from direct contact with components, drug product containers, closures, in-process materials, and drug products until the condition is corrected or determined by competent medical personnel not to jeopardize the safety or quality of drug products. All personnel shall be instructed to report to supervisory personnel any health conditions that may have an adverse effect on drug products.

211.34 Consultants

Consultants advising on the manufacture, processing, packing, or holding of drug products shall have sufficient education, training, and experience, or any combination thereof, to advise on the subject for which they are retained. Records shall be maintained stating the name, address, and qualifications of any consultants and the type of service they provide.

Subpart C—Buildings and Facilities

211.42 Design and construction features

(a) Any building or buildings used in the manufacture, processing, packing, or holding of a drug product shall be of suitable size, construction and location to facilitate cleaning, maintenance, and proper operations.

(b) Any such building shall have adequate space for the orderly placement of equipment and materials to prevent mix ups between different components, drug product containers, closures, labeling, in-process materials, or drug products, and to prevent contamination. The flow of components, drug product containers, closures, labeling, in-process materials, and drug products through the building or buildings shall be designed to prevent contamination.

(c) Operations shall be performed within specifically defined areas of adequate size. There shall be separate or defined areas or such other control systems for the firm's operations as are necessary to prevent contamination or mix ups during the course of the following procedures:

(1) Receipt, identification, storage, and withholding from use of components, drug product containers, closures, and labeling, pending the appropriate sampling, testing, or examination by the quality control unit before release for manufacturing or packaging

(2) Holding rejected components, drug product containers, closures, and labeling before disposition

(3) Storage of released components, drug product containers, closures, and labeling

(4) Storage of in-process materials

(5) Manufacturing and processing operations

(6) Packaging and labeling operations

(7) Quarantine storage before release of drug products

(8) Storage of drug products after release

(9) Control and laboratory operations

(10) Aseptic processing, which includes as appropriate:

(i) Floors, walls, and ceilings of smooth, hard surfaces that are easily cleanable

        (ii) Temperature and humidity controls

        (iii) An air supply filtered through high-efficiency particulate air filters under positive pressure, regardless of whether flow is laminar or no laminar;

        (iv) A system for monitoring environmental conditions

        (v) A system for cleaning and disinfecting the room and equipment to produce aseptic conditions

        (vi) A system for maintaining any equipment used to control the aseptic conditions.

(d) Operations relating to the manufacture, processing, and packing of penicillin shall be performed in facilities separate from those used for other drug products for human use.

211.44 Lighting

Adequate lighting shall be provided in all areas.

211.46 Ventilation, air filtration, air heating and cooling

(a) Adequate ventilation shall be provided.

(b) Equipment for adequate control over air pressure, micro-organisms, dust, humidity, and temperature shall be provided when appropriate for the manufacture, processing, packing, or holding of a drug product.

(c) Air filtration systems, including pre filters and particulate matter air filters, shall be used when appropriate on air supplies to production areas. If air is recirculated to production areas, measures shall be taken to control recirculation of dust from production. In areas where air contamination occurs during production, there shall be adequate exhaust systems or o their systems adequate to control contaminants.

(d) Air-handling systems for the manufacture, processing, and packing of penicillin shall be completely separate from those for other drug products for human use.

211.48 Plumbing

(a) Potable water shall be supplied under continuous positive pressure in a plumbing system free of defects that could contribute contamination to any drug product. Potable water shall meet the standards prescribed in the Environmental Protection Agency's Primary Drinking Water Regulations set forth in 40 CFR part 141. Water not meeting such standards shall not be permitted in the potable water system.

(b) Drains shall be of adequate size and, where connected directly to a sewer, shall be provided with an air break or other mechanical device to prevent back-siphonage.

211.50 Sewage and refuse

Sewage, trash, and other refuse in and from the building and immediate premises shall be disposed of in a safe and sanitary manner.

211.52 Washing and toilet facilities

Adequate washing facilities shall be provided, including hot and cold water, soap or detergent, air driers or single service towels, and clean toilet facilities easily accesible to working areas.

211.56 Sanitation

(a) Any building used in the manufacture, processing, packing, or holding of a drug product shall be maintained in a clean and sanitary condition, Any such building shall be free of infestation by rodents, birds, insects, and other vermin (other than laboratory animals).Trash and organic waste matter shall be held and disposed of in a timely and sanitary manner.

(b) There shall be written procedures assigning responsibility for sanitation and describing in sufficient detail the cleaning schedules, methods, equipment, and materials to be used in cleaning the buildings and facilities; such written procedures shall be followed.

(c) There shall be written procedures for use of suitable rodenticides, insecticides, fungicides, fumigating agents, and cleaning and sanitizing agents. Such written procedures shall be designed to prevent the contamination of equipment, components, drug product containers, closures, packaging, labeling materials, or drug products and shall be followed. Rodenticides, insecticides, and fungicides shall not be used unless registered and used in accordance with the Federal Insecticide, Fungicide, and Rodenticide Act (7 U.S.C.135).

(d) Sanitation procedures shall apply to work performed by contractors or temporary employees as well as work performed by full-time employees during the ordinary course of operations.

211.58 Maintenance

Any building used in the manufacture, processing, packing, or holding of a drug product shall be maintained in a good state of repair.

Subpart D—Equipment

211.63 Equipment design, size, and location

Equipment used in the manufacture, processing, packing, or holding of a drug product shall be of appropriate design, adequate size, and suitably located to facilitate operations for its intended use and for its cleaning and maintenance.

211.65 Equipment construction

(a) Equipment shall be constructed so that surfaces that contact components, in-process materials, or drug products shall not be reactive, additive, or absorptive so as to alter the safety, identity, strength, quality, or purity of the drug product beyond the official or other established requirements.

(b) Any substances required for operation, such as lubricants or coolants, shall not come into contact with components, drug product containers, closures, in-process materials, or drug products so as to alter the safety, identity, strength, quality, or purity of the drug product beyond the official or other established requirements.

211.67 Equipment cleaning and maintenance

(a) Equipment and utensils s hall be cleaned, maintained, and, as appropriate f or the nature of the drug, sanitized and/or sterilized at appropriate intervals to prevent malfunctions or contamination that would alter the safety, identity, strength, quality, or purity of the drug product beyond the official or other established requirements.

(b) Written procedures shall be established and followed for cleaning and maintenance of equipment, including utensils, used in the manufacture, processing, packing, or holding of a drug product. These procedures shall include, but are not necessarily limited to, the following:

(1) Assignment of responsibility for cleaning and maintaining equipment;

(2) Maintenance and cleaning schedules, including, where appropriate, sanitizing schedules;

(3) A description in sufficient detail of the methods, equipment, and materials used in cleaning and maintenance operations, and the methods of disassembling and reassembling equipment as necessary to assure proper cleaning and maintenance;

(4) Removal or obliteration of previous batch identification;

(5) Protection of clean equipment from contamination prior to use

(6) Inspection of equipment for cleanliness immediately before use.

(c) Records shall be kept of maintenance, cleaning, sanitizing, and inspection as specified in § 211.180 and §211.182.

211.68 Automatic, mechanical, and electronic equipment

(a) Automatic, mechanical, or electronic equipment or other types of equipment, including computers, or related systems that will perform a function satisfactorily, may be used in the manufacture, processing, packing, and holding of a drug product. If such equipment is so used, it shall be routinely calibrated, inspected, or checked according to a written program designed to assure proper performance. Written records of those calibration checks and inspections shall be maintained.

(b) Appropriate controls shall be exercised over computer or related systems to assure that changes in master production and control records or other records are instituted only by authorized personnel. Input to and output from the computer or related system of formulas or other records or data shall be checked for accuracy. The degree and frequency of input/output verification shall be based on the complexity and reliability of the computer or related system. A backup file of data entered into the computer or related syste..a shall be maintained except where certain data, such as calculations performed in connection with laboratory analysis, are eliminated by computerization or other automated processes. In such instances a written record of the program shall be maintained along with appropriate validation data. Hard copy or alternative systems, such as duplicates, tapes, or microfilm, designed to assure that backup data are exact and complete and that it is secure from alteration, inadvertent erasures, or loss shall be maintained.

211.72 Filters

Filters for liquid filtration used in the manufacture, processing, or packing of injectable drug products intended for human use shall not release fibers into such products. Fiber-releasing filters may be used when it is not possible to manufacture such products without the use of these filters. If use of a fiber-releasing filter is necessary, an additional non fiber-releasing filter having a maximum nominal pore size rating of 0.2 micron (0.45 micron if the manufacturing conditions so dictate) shall subsequently be used to reduce the content of particles in the injectable drug product. The use of an asbestos-containing filter is prohibited.

Subpart E—Control of Components and Drug Product Containers and Closures

211.80 General requirements

(a) There shall be written procedures describing in sufficient detail the receipt, identification, storage, handling, sampling, testing, and approval or rejection of components and drug product containers and closures; such written procedures shall be followed.

(b) Components and drug product containers and closures shall at all times be handled and stored in a manner to prevent contamination.

(c) Bagged or boxed components of drug product containers, or closures shall be stored off the floor and suitably spaced to permit cleaning and inspection.

(d) Each container or grouping of containers for components or drug product containers, or closures shall be identified with a distinctive code for each lot in each shipment received.

211.82 Receipt and storage of untested components, drug product containers, and closures

(a) Upon receipt and before acceptance, each container or grouping of containers of components, drug product containers, and closures shall be examined visually for appropriate labeling as to contents, container damage or broken seals, and contamination.

(b) Components, drug product containers, and closures shall be stored under quarantine until they have been tested or examined, whichever is appropriate, and released. Storage within the area shall conform to the requirements of § 211.80.

211.84 Testing and approval or rejection of components, drug product containers, and closures

(a) Each lot of components, drug product containers, and closures shall be withheld from use until the lot has been sampled, tested, or examined, as appropriate, and released for use by the quality control unit.

(b) Representative samples of each shipment of each lot shall be collected for testing or examination. The number of containers to be sampled, and the amount of material to be taken from each container, shall be based upon appropriate criteria such as statistical criteria for component variability, confidence levels, and degree of precision desired, the past quality history of the supplier, and the quantity needed for analysis and reserve where required by § 211.170.

(c) Samples shall be collected in accordance with the following procedures;

(1) The containers of components selected shall be cleaned when necessary in a manner to prevent introduction of contaminants into the component.

(2) The containers shall be opened, sampled, and resealed in a manner designed to prevent contamination of their contents and contamination of other components, drug product containers, or closures.

(3) Sterile equipment and aseptic sampling techniques shall be used when necessary.

(4) If it is necessary to sample a component from the top, middle, and bottom of its container, such sample subdivisions shall not be composited for testing.

(5) Sample containers shall be identified .

(6) Containers from which samples have been taken shall be marked to show that samples have been removed from them.

(d) Samples shall be examined and tested as follows:

(1) At least one test shall be conducted to verify the identity of each component of a drug product. Specific identity tests, if they exist, shall be used.

(2) Each component shall be tested for conformity with all appropriate written specifications for purity, strength, and quality. In lieu of such testing by the manufacturer, a report of analysis may be accepted from the supplier of a component, provided that at least one specific identity test is conducted on such component by the manufacturer, and provided that the manufacturer establishes the reliability of the supplier's analyses through appropriate validation of the supplier's test results at appropriate intervals.

(3) Containers and closures shall be tested for conformity with all appropriate written specifications. In lieu of such testing by the manufacturer, a certificate of testing may be accepted from the supplier, provided that at least a visual identification is conducted on such containers/closures by the manufacturer and provided that the manufacturer establishes the reliability of the supplier's test results through appropriate validation of the supplier's test results at appropriate intervals.

(4) When appropriate, components shall be microscopically examined.

(5) Each lot of a component, drug product container, or closure that is liable to contamination with filth, insect infestation, or other extraneous adulterant shall be examined against established specifications for such contamination.

(6) Each lot of a component, drug product container, or closure with potential for microbiological contamination that is objectionable in view of its intended use shall be subjected to microbiological tests before use.

(e)   Any lot of components, drug product containers, or closures that meets the appropriate written specifications of identity, strength, quality, and purity and related tests under paragraph (d) of this section may be approved and released for use. Any lot of such material that does not meet such specifications shall be rejected.

211.86 Use of approved components, drug product containers, and closures

Components, drug product containers, and closures approved for use shall be rotated so that the oldest approved stock is used first. Deviation from this requirement is permitted if such deviation is temporary and appropriate.

211.87 Retesting of approved components, drug product containers, and closures

Components, drug product containers, and closures shall be retested or reexamined, as appropriate, for identity, strength, quality, and purity and approved or rejected by the quality control unit in accordance with § 211.84 as necessary, e.g., after storage for long periods or after exposure to air, heat or other conditions that might adversely affect the component, drug product container, or closure.

211.89 Rejected components, drug product containers, and closure

Rejected components, drug product containers, and closures shall be identified and controlled under a quarantine system designed to prevent their use in manufacturing or processing operations for which they are unsuitable.

211.94 Drug product containers and closures

(a) Drug product containers and closures shall not be reactive, additive, or absorptive so as to alter the safety, identity, strength, quality, or purity of the drug beyond the official or established requirements.

(b) Container closure systems shall provide adequate protection against foreseeable external factors in storage and use that can cause deterioration or contamination of the drug product.

(c) Drug product containers and closures shall be clean and, where indicated by the nature of the drug, sterilized and processed to remove pyrogenic properties to assure that they are suitable for their intended use. Such depyrogenation processes shall be validated.

(d) Standards or specifications, methods of testing, and, where indicated, methods of cleaning, sterilizing, and processing to remove pyrogenic properties shall be written and followed for drug product containers and closures.

Subpart F—Production and Process Controls

211.100 Written procedures; deviations:

(a) There shall be written procedures for production and process control designed to assure that the drug products have the identity, strength, quality, and purity they purport or are represented to possess.

(b) Written production and process control procedures shall be followed in the execution of the various production and process control functions and shall be documented at the time of performance. Any deviation from the written procedures shall be recorded and justified.

211.101 Charge-in of components

Written production and control procedures shall include the following, which are designed to assure that the drug products produced have the identity, strength, quality, and purity they

purport or are represented to possess:

(a) The batch shall be formulated with the intent to provide not less than 100 percent of the labeled or established amount of active ingredient.

(b) Components for drug product manufacturing shall be weighed, measured, or subdivided as appropriate.

(c) Weighing, measuring, or subdividing operations for components shall be adequately supervised.

(d) Each component shall either be added to the batch by one person and verified by a second person or, if the components are added by automated equipment under § 211.68, only verified by one person.

211.103 Calculation of yield

Actual yields and percentages of theoretical yield shall be determined at the conclusion of each appropriate phase of manufacturing, processing, packaging, or holding of the drug product. Such calculations shall either be performed by one person and independently verified by a second person, or, if the yield is calculated by automated equipment under § 211.68, be independently verified by one person.

211.105 Equipment identification

(a) All compounding and storage containers, processing lines, and major equipment used during the production of a batch of a drug product shall be properly identified at all times to indicate their contents and, when necessary, the phase of processing of the batch.

(b) Major equipment shall be identified by a distinctive identification number or code that shall be recorded in the batch production record to show the specific equipment used in the manufacture of each batch of a drug product. In cases where only one of a particular type of equipment exists in a manufacturing facility, the name of the equipment may be used in lieu of a distinctive identification number or code.

211.110 Sampling and testing of inprocess materials and drug products

(a) To assure batch uniformity and integrity of drug products, written procedures shall be established and followed that describe the in-process controls, and tests, or examinations to be conducted on appropriate samples of in-process materials of each batch. Such control procedures shall be established to monitor the output and to validate the performance of those manufacturing processes that may be responsible for causing variability in the characteristics of in-process material and the drug product.

(b) Valid in-process specifications for such characteristics shall be consistent with drug product final specifications and shall be derived from previous acceptable process average and process variability estimates where possible and determined by the application of suitable statistical procedures where appropriate.

Examination and testing of samples shall assure that the drug product and in-process material conform to specifications.

(c) In-process materials shall be tested for identity, strength, quality, and purity as appropriate, and approved or rejected by the quality control unit, during the production process.

(d) Rejected in-process materials shall be identified and controlled under a quarantine system designed to prevent their use in manufacturing or processing operations for which they are unsuitable.

211.111 Time limitations on production

When appropriate, time limits for the completion of each phase of production shall be established to assure the quality of the drug product. Deviation from established time limits may be acceptable if such deviation does not compromise the quality of the drug product. Such deviation shall be justified and documented.

211.113 Control of microbiological contamination

(a) Appropriate written procedures designed to prevent objectionable microorganisms in drug products noestablished and followed.

(b) Appropriate written procedures, designed to prevent microbiological contamination of drug products purporting to be sterile, shall be established and followed. Such procedures shall include validation of all aseptic and sterilization processes.

211.115 Reprocessing:

(a) Written procedures shall be established and followed prescribing a system for reprocessing batches that do not conform to standards or specifications and the steps to be taken to insure that the reprocessed batches will conform with all established standards, specifications, and characteristics.

(b) Reprocessing shall not be performed without the review and approval of the quality control unit.

Subpart G—Packaging and Labeling Control

211.122 Materials examination and usage criteria

(a) There shall be written procedures describing in sufficient detail the receipt, identification, storage, handling, sampling, examination, and/or testing of labeling and packaging materials.

(b) Any labeling or packaging materials meeting appropriate written specifications may be approved and released for use.

(c) Records shall be maintained for each shipment received of each different labeling and packaging material indicating receipt, examination or testing, and whether accepted or rejected.

(d) Labels and other labeling materials for each different drug product, strength, dosage form, or quantity of contents shall be stored separately with suitable identification.

(e) Obsolete and outdated labels, labeling, and other packaging materials shall be destroyed.

(f) Use of gang-printed labeling for different drug products, or different strengths or net contents of the same drug product, is prohibited unless the labeling from gang-printed sheets is adequately differentiated by size, shape, or color.

(g) If cut labeling is used, packaging and labeling operations shall include one of the following special control procedures:

(1) Dedication of labeling and packaging lines to each different strength of each different drug product.

(2) Use of appropriate electronic or electromechanical equipment to conduct a 100-percent examination for correct labeling during or after completion of finishing operations; or

(3) Use of visual inspection to conduct a 100-percent examination for correct labeling during or after completion of finishing operations for hand applied labeling.

(h) Printing devices on, or associated with, manufacturing lines used to imprint labeling upon the drug product unit label or case shall be monitored to assure that all imprinting conforms to the print specified in the batch production record.

211.125 Labeling issuance

(a) Strict control shall be exercised over labeling issued for use in drug product labeling operations.

(b) Labeling materials issued for a batch shall be carefully examined for identity and conformity to the labeling specified in the master or batch production records.

(c) Procedures shall be used to reconcile the quantities of labeling issued used, and returned, and shall require evaluation of discrepancies found between the quantity of drug product finished and the quantity of labeling issued when such discrepancies are outside narrow preset limits based on historical operating data.

(d) All excess labeling bearing lot or control numbers shall be destroyed.

(e) Returned labeling shall be maintained and stored in a manner to prevent mix ups and provide proper identification.

(f) Procedures shall be written describing in sufficient detail the control procedures employed for the issuance of labeling; such written procedures shall be followed.

211.130 Packaging and labeling operations

Written procedures shall be followed. These procedures shall incorporate the following features:

(a) Prevention of mix ups and cross contamination by physical or spatial separation from operations on other drug products.

(b) Identification and handling of filled drug product containers that are set aside and held in unlabeled condition for future labeling operations to preclude mislabeling of individual containers, lots, or portions of lots. Identification need not be applied to each individual container but shall be sufficient to determine name, strength, quantity of contents, and lot or control number of each container.

(c) Identification of the drug product with a lot or control number that permits determination of the history of the manufacture and control of the batch.

(d) Examination of packaging and labeling materials for suitability and correctness before packaging operations, and documentation of such examination in the batch production record.

(e) Inspection of the packaging and labeling facilities immediately before use to assure that all drug products have been removed from previous operations.

211.132 Tamper-evident packaging requirements for over-the-counter (OTC) human drug products

(a) An OTC drug product (except a dermatological, dentifrice, insulin, or lozenge product) for retail sale that is not packaged in a tamper-resistant package or that is not properly labeled under this section is adulterated under section 501 of the act or misbranded under section 502 of the act, or both.

(b) **Requirements for tamper-evident package**

(1) Each manufacturer and packer who packages an OTC drug product (except a dermatological, dentifrice, insulin, or lozenge product) for retail sale shall package the product in a tamper-evident package, if this product is accessible to the public while held for sale.

(2) In addition to the tamper-evident packaging feature described in paragraph (b)(1) of this section, any two piece, hard gelatin capsule covered by this section must be sealed using an acceptable tamper-evident technology.

(c) **Labeling:** In order to alert consumers to the specific tamper-evident feature(s) used, each retail package of an OTC drug product covered by this section is required to bear a statement that: (i) Identifies all tamper-evident feature(s) and any capsule sealing technologies.

(ii) Is prominently placed on the package; and

(iii) Is so placed that it will be unaffected if the tamper-evident feature of the package is breached or missing, table tamper-evident technology.

211.134 Drug product inspection

(a) Packaged and labeled products shall be examined during finishing operations to provide assurance that containers and packages in the lot have the correct label.

(b) A representative sample of units shall be collected at the completion of finishing operations and shall be visually examined for correct labeling.

(c) Results of these examinations shall be recorded in the batch production or control records.

211.137 Expiration dating

(a) To assure that a drug product meets applicable standards of identity, strength, quality, and purity at the time of use, it shall bear an expiration date determined by appropriate stability testing described in § 211.166.

(b) Expiration dates shall be related to any storage conditions stated on the labeling, as determined by stability studies described in § 211.166.

(c) If the drug product is to be reconstituted at the time of dispensing, its labeling shall bear expiration information for both the reconstituted and un reconstituted drug products.

(d) Expiration dates shall appear on labeling.

Subpart H—Holding and Distribution

211.142 Warehousing procedures

(a) Quarantine of drug products before release by the quality control unit.

(b) Storage of drug products under appropriate conditions of temperature, humidity, and light so that the identity, strength, quality, and purity of the drug products are not affected.

211.150 Distribution procedures.

(a) A procedure whereby the oldest approved stock of a drug product is distributed first.

(b) A system by which the distribution of each lot of drug product can be readily determined to facilitate its recall if necessary.

Subpart I—Laboratory Controls

211.160 General requirements

(a) The establishment of any specifications, standards, sampling plans, test procedures, or other laboratory control mechanisms required by this subpart, including any change in such specifications, standards, sampling plans, test procedures, or other laboratory control mechanisms, shall be drafted by the appropriate organizational unit and reviewed and approved by the quality control unit.

(b) Laboratory controls shall include the establishment of scientifically sound and appropriate specifications, standards, sampling plans, and test procedures designed to assure thatcomponents, drug product containers, closures, in-process materials, labeling, and drug products conform to appropriate standards of identity, strength, quality, and purity.

211.165 Testing and release for distribution

(a) For each batch of drug product, there shall be appropriate laboratory determination of satisfactory conformance to final specifications for the drug product, including the identity and strength of each active ingredient, prior to release.

(b) There shall be appropriate laboratory testing, as necessary, of each batch of drug product required to be free of objectionable microorganisms.

(c) Any sampling and testing plans shall be described in written procedures that shall include the method of sampling and the number of units per batch to be tested; such written procedure shall be followed.

(d) Acceptance criteria for the sampling and testing conducted by the quality control unit shall be adequate to assure that batches of drug products meet each appropriate specification and appropriate statistical quality control criteria as a condition for their approval and release.

(e) The accuracy, sensitivity, specificity, and reproducibility of test methods employed by the firm shall be established and documented.

(f) Drug products failing to meet established standards or specifications and any other relevant quality control criteria shall be rejected.

211.166 Stability testing

(a) The written program shall be followed and shall include:

(1) Sample size and test intervals based on statistical criteria for each attribute examined to assure valid estimates of stability;

(2) Storage conditions for samples retained for testing;

(3) Reliable, meaningful, and specific test methods;

(4) Testing of the drug product in the same container-closure system as that in which the drug product is marketed.

(5) Testing of drug products for reconstitution at the time of dispensing (as directed in the labeling) as well as after they are reconstituted.

(b) An adequate number of batches of each drug product shall be tested to determine an appropriate expiration date and a record of such data shall be maintained. Accelerated studies, combined with basic stability information on the components, drug products, and container-closure system, may be used to support tentative expiration dates provided full shelf life studies are not available and are being conducted.

211.167 Special testing requirements

(a) For each batch of drug product purporting to be sterile and/or pyrogen free, there shall be appropriate laboratory testing to determine conformance to such requirements.

(b) For each batch of ophthalmic ointment, there shall be appropriate testing to determine conformance to specifications regarding the presence of foreign particles and harsh or abrasive substances.

(c) For each batch of controlled-release dosage form, there shall be appropriate laboratory testing to determine conformance to the specifications for the rate of release of each active ingredient.

211.170 Reserve samples

(a) An appropriately identified reserve sample that is representative of each lot in each shipment of each active ingredient shall be retained. The reserve sample consists of at least twice the quantity necessary for all tests required to determine whether the active ingredient meets its established specifications, except for sterility and pyrogen testing.

(b) An appropriately identified reserve sample that is representative of each lot or batch of drug product shall be retained and stored under conditions consistent with product labeling.

211.173 Laboratory animals

Animals used in testing components, in-process materials, or drug products for compliance with established specifications shall be maintained and controlled in a manner that assures their suitability for their intended use. They shall be identified, and adequate records shall be maintained showing the history of their use.

211.176 Penicillin contamination

If a reasonable possibility exists that a non-penicillin drug product has been exposed to cross-contamination with penicillin, the non-penicillin drug product shall be tested for the presence of penicillin. Such drug product shall not be marketed if detectable levels are found when tested according to procedures specified in 'Procedures for Detecting and Measuring Penicillin Contamination in Drugs,' which is incorporated by reference.

Subpart J—Records and Reports

211.180 General requirements

(a) Any production, control, or distribution record that is required to be maintained in complia nce with this part and is specifically associated with a batch of a drug product shall be retained for at least 1 year after the expiration date of the batch or, in the case of certain OTC drug products lacking expiration dating because they meet the criteria for exemption under§ 211.137, 3 years after distribution of the batch.

(b) Records shall be maintained for all components, drug product containers, closures, and labeling for at least 1 year after the expiration date or, in the case of certain OTC drug products lacking expiration dating because they meet the criteria for exemption under § 211.137, 3 years after distribution of the last lot of drug product incorporating the component or using the container, closure, or labeling.

(c) All records required under this part, or copies of such records, shall be readily available for authorized inspection during the retention period at the establishment where the activities described in such records occurred.

(d) Records required under this part may be retained either as original records or as true copies such as photocopies, microfilm, microfiche, or other accurate reproductions of the original records.

(e) Written records required by this part shall be maintained so that data therein can be used for evaluating, at least annually, the quality standards of each drug product to determine the need for changes in drug product specifications or manufacturing or control procedures.

211.182 Equipment cleaning and use log

A written record of major equipment cleaning, maintenance (except routine maintenance such as lubrication and adjustments), and use shall be included in individual equipment logs that show the date, time, product, and lot number of each batch processed. The persons performing and double-checking the cleaning and maintenance shall date and sign or initial the log indicating that the work was performed. Entries in the log shall be in chronological order.

211.184 Component, drug product container, closure, and labeling records

These records shall include the following:

(a) The identity and quantity of each shipment of each lot of components, drug product containers, closures, and labeling; the name of the supplier; the supplier's lot number(s) if known; the receiving code as specified in § 211.80; and the date of receipt.

(b) The results of any test or examination performed and the conclusions derived there from.

(c) An individual inventory record of each component, drug product container, and closure and, for each component, a reconciliation of the use of each lot of such component.

(d) Documentation of the examination and review of labels and labeling for conformity with established specifications in accord with §§ 211.122(c) and 211.130(c).

(e) The disposition of rejected components, drug product containers, closure, and labeling.

211.186 Master production and control records

(a) To assure uniformity from batch to batch, master production and control records for each drug product, including each batch size thereof, shall be prepared, dated, and signed by one person and independently checked, dated, and signed by a second person.

(b) Master production and control records shall include:

(1) The name and strength of the product and a description of the dosage form;

(2) The name and weight or measure of each active ingredient per dosage unit or per unit of weight or measure of the drug product and a statement of the total weight or measure of any dosage unit;

(3) A complete list of components designated by names or codes sufficiently specific to indicate any special quality characteristic.

(4) An accurate statement of the weight or measure of each component, using the same weight system (metric, avoirdupois, or apothecary) for each component;

(5) A statement concerning any calculated excess of component;

(6) A statement of theoretical weight or measure at appropriate phases of processing;

(7) A statement of theoretical yield, including the maximum and minimum percentages of theoretical yield beyond which investigation according to § 211.192 is required;

(8) A description of the drug product containers, closures, and packaging materials, including a specimen or copy of each label and all other labeling signed and dated by the person or persons responsible for approval of such labeling;

(9) Complete manufacturing and control instructions, sampling and testing procedures, specifications, special notations, and precautions to be followed.

211.188 Batch production and control records

These records shall include:

(a) An accurate reproduction of the appropriate master production or control record, checked for accuracy, dated, and signed.

(b) Documentation that each significant step in the manufacture, processing, packing, or holding of the batch was accomplished, including.

(1) Dates

(2) Identity of individual major equipment and lines used

(3) Specific identification of each batch of component or in-process material used

(4) Weights and measures of components used in the course of processing

(5) In-process and laboratory control results

(6) Inspection of the packaging and labeling area before and after use

(7) A statement of the actual yield and a statement of the percentage of theoretical yield at appropriate phases of processing

(8) Complete labeling control records including specimens or copies of all labeling used

(9) Description of drug product containers and closures

(10) Any sampling performeds

211.192 Production record review

All drug product production and control records, including those for packaging and labeling, shall be reviewed and approved by the quality control unit to determine compliance with all established, approved written procedures before a batch is released or distributed.

Any unexplained discrepancy or the failure of a batch or any of its components to meet any of its specifications shall be thoroughly investigated.

211.194 Laboratory records

(a) Laboratory records shall include complete data derived from all tests necessary to assure compliance with established specifications and standards, including examinations and assays, as follows:

(1) A description of the sample received for testing with identification of source, quantity, lot number or other distinctive

code, date sample was taken, and date sample was received for testing.

(2) A statement of each method used in the testing of the sample.

(3) A statement of the weight or measure of sample used for each test, where appropriate.

(4) A complete record of all data secured in the course of each test, including all graphs, charts, and spectra from laboratory instrumentation, properly identified to show the specific component, drug product container, closure, in-process material, or drug product, and lot tested.

(5) A record of all calculations performed in connection with the test, including units of measure, conversion factors, and equivalency factors.

(6) A statement of the results of tests and how the results compare with established standards of identity, strength, quality, and purity for the component, drug product container, closure, in-process material, or drug product tested.

(7) The initials or signature of the person who performs each test and the date(s) the tests were performed.

(8) The initials or signature of a second person showing that the original records have been reviewed for accuracy, completeness, and compliance with established standards.

(b) Complete records shall be maintained of any modification of an established method employed in testing.

(c) Complete records shall be maintained of any testing and standardization of laboratory reference standards, reagents, and standard solutions.

(d) Complete records shall be maintained of the periodic calibration of laboratory instruments, apparatus, gauges, and recording devices required by § 211.160(b)(4).

(e) Complete records shall be maintained of all stability testing performed in accordance with § 211.166.

211.196 Distribution records

Distribution records shall contain the name and strength of the product and description of the dosage form, name and address of the consignee, date and quantity shipped, and lot or control number of the drug product.

211.198 Complaint files

(a) Written procedures describing the handling of all written and oral complaints regarding a drug product shall be established and followed.

(b) A written record of each complaint shall be maintained in a file designated for drug product complaints.

Subpart K—Returned and Salvaged Drug Products

211.204 Returned drug products

Returned drug products shall be identified as such and held. If the conditions under which returned drug products have been held, stored, or shipped before or during their return, or if the condition of the drug product, its container, carton, or labeling, as a result of storage or shipping, casts doubt on the safety, identity, strength, quality or purity of the drug product, the returned drug product shall be destroyed unless examination, testing, or other investigations prove the drug product meets appropriate standards of safety, identity, strength, quality, or purity. A drug product may be reprocessed provided the subsequent drug product meets appropriate standards, specifications, and characteristics. Records of returned drug products shall be maintained and shall include the name and label potency of the drug product dosage form, lot number (or control number or batch number), reason for the return, quantity returned, date of disposition, and ultimate disposition of the returned drug product

211.208 Drug product salvaging

Drug products that have been subjected to improper storage conditions including extremes in temperature, humidity, smoke, fumes, pressure, age, or radiation due to natural disasters, fires, accidents, or equipment failures shall not be salvaged and returned to the marketplace. Whenever there is a question whether drug products have been subjected to such conditions, salvaging operations may be conducted only if there is (a) evidence from laboratory tests and assays (including animal feeding studies where applicable) that the drug products meet all applicable standards of identity, strength, quality , and purity and (b) evidence from inspection of the premises that the drug products and their associated packaging were not subjected to improper storage conditions as a result of the disaster or accident. Organoleptic examinations shall be acceptable only as supplemental evidence that the drug products meet appropriate standards of identity, strength, quality, and purity. Records including name, lot number, and disposition shall be maintained for drug products subject to this section.

REVIEW QUESTIONS

ESSAY QUESTIONS

1. Write about USFDA guidelines for manufacturing of pharmaceuticals?

2. Write the current good manufacturing practice for finished pharmaceuticals as per CFR 21 part 210 and 211 of USFDA ?

3. Write the Good manufacturing practices for premises and materials as per Schedule M?

4. Write the Good manufacturing Requirements of Plants and Equipments as per Schedule M?

5. Write about Master Formula records and Batch processing Record?

6. Write the specific requirements for manufacture of sterile products as per Schedule M?

7. Write the specific requirements for manufacture of oral solid dosage forms as per Schedule M?

SHORT ANSWER QUESTIONS

1. Write the significance of Good Manufacturing Practice in Pharmaceutical Industry?

2. Write an overview of GMP and cGMP?

3. Write the specific requirements for manufacture of metered-dose inhalers as per Schedule M?

4. Write the specific requirements for manufacture of oral liquids as per Schedule M?

5. Write the specific requirements for manufacture of topical products as per Schedule M

6. Write short notes on Master Formula records?

7. Write about Batch processing Record ?

Chapter 8

INTRODUCTION TO VALIDATION

8.1 PROCESS VALIDATION

Process Validation is the means of ensuring, and providing documentary evidence that processes (within their specified design parameters) are capable of repeatedly and reliably producing a finished product of the required quality. Any manufacturing process will involve a number of factors that may affect product quality. These factors will be identified during the development of a product and will facilitate process optimization studies. On completion of development and optimization, Process Validation provides a structured way of assessing methodically the factors that impact on the final product. Pharmaceutical process validation should cover all the critical elements in a manufacturing process for a pharmaceutical product, from development of the process through to final validation at the production scale. While it is recognised that the term validation is intended to apply to the final verification at the production scale (typically 3 production batches), the guidance presented here is intended to encompass the information that should routinely be included in the marketing authorisation application.

USFDA defined process validation as "Establishing documented evidence, which provides a high degree of assurance that a specific process will consistently produce a product meeting its pre determined specifications and quality attributes".

8.2 PRE-REQUISITES FOR PROCESS VALIDATION

Before process validation can be started, manufacturing equipment and control instruments as well as the formulation mustbe qualified. The Information on a pharmaceutical product should be studied in detail and qualified at the development stage, i.e., before an application for marketing authorization is submitted. This involves studies on the compatibility of active ingredients and recipients, and of final drug product and packaging materials, stability studies, etc. Other aspects of manufacture must be validated including critical services (water, air, nitrogen, power supply, etc.) and supporting operations such as equipment cleaning and sanitation of premises. Proper training and motivation of personnel are prerequisites to successful validation.

8.3 THE PHARMACEUTICAL PROCESS EQUIPMENT

The key idea of validation is to provide a high level of documented evidence that the equipment and the process conform to a written standard. The level (or depth) is dictated by the complexity of the system or equipment. The validation package must provide the necessary information and test procedures required to provide that the system and process meet specified requirements. Validation of pharmaceutical process equipment involves the following:

1. **Installation Qualification:** This ensures that all major processing and packaging equipment, and ancillary systems are in conformity with installation specification, equipment manuals schematics and engineering drawing. It verifies that the equipment has been installed in accordance with manufacturers recommendation in a proper manner and placed in an environment suitable for its intended purpose.

2. **Operational Qualification:** This is done to provide a high degree of assurance that the equipment functions as intended. Operational qualification should be conducted in two stages:

   Component Operational Qualification, of which calibration can be considered a large part.

   System Operational Qualification to determine if the entire system operates as an integrated whole.

3. **Process Performance Qualification:** This verifies that the system is repeatable and is consistently producing a quality product.

The **Process validation activities** can be described in three stages.

Stage 1 – Process Design: The commercial process is defined during this stage based on knowledge gained through development and scale-up activities.

Stage 2 – Process Qualification: During this stage, the process design is confirmed as being capable of reproducible commercial manufacturing.

Stage 3 – Continued Process Verification: Ongoing assurance is gained during routine production that the process remains in a state of control.

8.4 PHASES OF PROCESS VALIDATION

The activities relating to validation studies may be classified into three phases:

Phase 1:

Pre-Validation Phase or the Qualification Phase, which covers all activities relating to product research and development, formulation, pilot batch studies, scale-up studies, transfer of technology to commercial scale batches, establishing stability conditions, storage and handling of in-process and finished dosage forms, equipment qualification, installation qualification, master production documents, operational qualification, process capability.

Phase 2:

Process Validation Phase (Process Qualification phase) designed to verify that all established limits of the critical process parameters are valid and that satisfactory products can be produced even under the "worst case" conditions.

Phase 3:

Validation Maintenance Phase requiring frequent review of all process related documents, including validation audit reports to assure that there have been no changes, deviations, failures, modifications to the production process, and that all standard operating procedures have been followed, including Change Control procedures. At this stage the validation team also assures that there have been no changes/ deviations that should have resulted in requalification and revalidation.

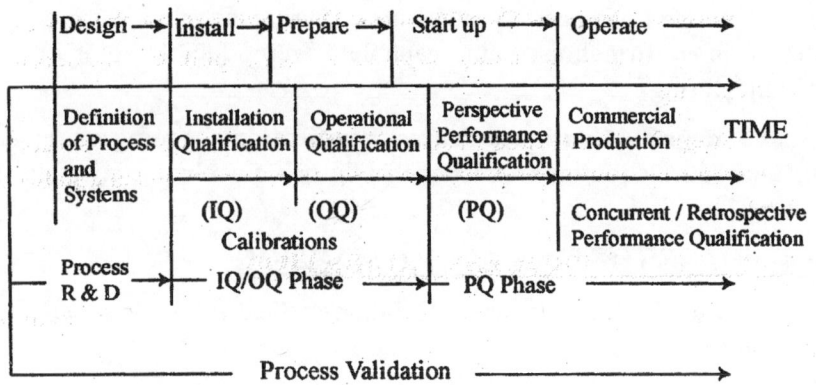

Fig.1: General view of process validation

8.5 VALIDATION PROTOCOL

The validation protocol provides a synopsis of what is hoped to be accomplished. The protocol should list the selected process and control parameters, state the number of batches to be included in the study, and specify how the data, once assembled, will be treated for relevance. The date of approval by the validation team should also be noted. In the case where a protocol is altered or modified after its approval, appropriate reasoning for such a change must be documented.

The validation protocol should be numbered, signed and dated, and should contain as a minimum the following information:

1. Title

2. Objective & Scope

3. Responsibility

4. Protocol Approval

5. Validation Team

6. Product Composition

7. Process Flow Chart

8. Manufacturing Process

9. Review of Equipments / Utilities

10. Review of Raw Materials and Packing Materials

11. Review of Analytical and Batch Manufacturing Records

12. Review of Batch Quantities for Validation (Raw Materials)

13. Review of Batch Quantities for Validation (Packing Materials)

14. Review of Process Parameters

15. Validation Procedure

16. Sampling Location

17. Documentation

18. Acceptance Criteria

19. Summary

20. Conclusion

8.6 THE VALIDATION REPORT

A written report should be available after completion of the validation. If found acceptable, it should be approved and authorized (signed and dated).

The report should include at least the following:

- Title and objective of study,
- Reference to protocol,
- Details of material,
- Equipment,

- Programmes and cycles used,

- Details of procedures and test methods,

- Results (compared with acceptance criteria) and

- Recommendations on the limit and criteria to be applied on future basis.

8.7 DOCUMENTATION

Documentation at each stage of the process validation lifecycle is essential for effective communication in complex, lengthy, and multidisciplinary projects. Documentation is important so that knowledge gained about a product and process is accessible and comprehensible to others involved in each stage of the lifecycle. In addition to being a fundamental tenet of following the scientific method, information transparency and accessibility are essential so that organizational units responsible and accountable for the process can make informed, science-based decisions that ultimately support the release of a product to commerce.

8.8 TYPES OF PROCESS VALIDATION

Depending on when it is performed in relation to production, validation can be prospective, concurrent, retrospective or revalidation (repeated validation).

PROSPECTIVE VALIDATION

In Prospective Validation, the validation protocol is executed before the process is put into commercial use. During the product development phase the production process should be broken down into individual steps. Each step should be evaluated on the basis of experience or theoretical considerations to determine the critical parameters that may affect the quality of the finished product. A series of experiments should be designed to determine the criticality of these factors. Each experiment should be planned and documented fully in an authorized protocol. All equipment, production environment and the analytical testing methods to be used should have been fully validated. Master batch documents can be prepared only after the critical parameters of the process have been identified and machine settings, component specifications and environmental conditions have been determined.

It is generally considered acceptable that three consecutive batches/runs within the finally agreed parameters, giving product of the desired quality would constitute a proper validation of the process. It is a confirmation on the commercial three batches before marketing. Upon completion of the review, recommendations should be made on the extent of monitoring and the in-process controls necessary for routine production. These should be incorporated into the batch manufacturing and packaging record or into appropriate standard operating procedures. Limits, frequencies and actions to be taken in the event of the limits being exceeded should be specified.

It may be possible and acceptable in particular circumstances for a manufacturer that uses the same process for several related products to develop a scientifically sound validation plan for that process rather than different plans for each product manufactured by that process. The matrix approach generally means a plan to conduct process validation on different strengths of the same product, whereas the "family" approach means a plan to conduct process validation on different products manufactured with the same processes using the same equipment.

The validation process using these approaches must include batches of different strengths or products which should be selected to represent the worst case conditions or scenarios to demonstrate that the process is consistent for all strengths or products involved.

CONCURRENT VALIDATION

Concurrent validation is carried out during normal production. This method is effective only if the development stage has resulted in a proper understanding of the fundamentals of the process. The first three production-scale batches must be monitored as comprehensively as possible. The nature and specifications of subsequent in-process and final tests are based on the evaluation of the results of such monitoring. Concurrent validation together with a trend analysis including stability should be carried out to an appropriate extent throughout the life of the product.

Concurrent validation may be the practical approach under certain circumstances. Examples of these may be when:

- A previously validated process is being transferred to a third party contract manufacturer or to another manufacturing site.

- The product is a different strength of a previously validated product with the same ratio of active/inactive ingredients.

- The number of lots evaluated under the Retrospective Validation were not sufficient to obtain a high degree of assurance demonstrating that the process is fully under control.

- The number of batches produced are limited (e.g. orphan drugs).

- Process with low production volume per batch (e.g. radiopharmaceuticals, anticancer).

- Process of manufacturing urgently needed drugs due to shortage (or absence) of supply.

It is important in these cases however, that the systems and equipment to be used have been fully validated previously. The justification for conducting concurrent validation must be documented and the protocol must be approved by the validation team. A report should be prepared and approved prior to the sale of each batch and a final report should be prepared and approved after the completion of all concurrent batches. It is generally considered acceptable that a minimum of three consecutive batches within the finally agreed parameters, giving the product the desired quality would constitute a proper validation of the process.

RETROSPECTIVE VALIDATION

Retrospective validation involves the examination of past experience of production on the assumption that composition, procedures, and equipment remain unchanged; such experience and the results of in process and final control tests are then evaluated. Recorded difficult and failures in production are analyzed to determine the limits of process parameters. A trend analysis may be conducted to determine the extent to which the process parameters are within the permissible range.

Retrospective validation is obviously not a quality assurance measure in itself, and should never be applied to new processes or products. It may be considered in special circumstances only, e.g. when validation requirements are first introduced in a company. Retrospective validation may then be useful in establishing the priorities for the validation programme. If the results of a retrospective validation are positive, this indicated that the process is not in need of immediate attention and may be validated in accordance with the normal schedule. For tablets which have been compressed under individual pressure-sensitive cells, and with qualified equipment, retrospective validation is the most comprehensive test of the overall manufacturing process of this dosage form. On the other hand, it should not be applied in the manufacture of sterile products.

Retrospective validation is only acceptable for well established detailed processes that include operational limits for each critical step of the process and will be inappropriate where there have been recent changes in the formulation of the product, operating procedures, equipment and facility.

The source of data for retrospective validation should include amongst others, batch documents, process control charts, maintenance log books, process capability studies, finished product test results, including trend analyses, and stability results.For the purpose of retrospective validation studies, it is considered acceptable that data from a minimum of ten consecutive batches produced be utilized. When less than ten batches are available, it is considered that the data are not sufficient to demonstrate retrospectively that the process is fully under control. In such cases the study should be supplemented with data generated with concurrent or prospective validation.

Some of the essential elements for Retrospective Validation are

- Batches manufactured for a defined period (minimum of 10 last consecutive batches).
- Number of lots released per year.
- Batch size/strength/manufacturer/year/period.
- Master manufacturing/packaging documents.

- Current specifications for active materials/finished products.
- List of process deviations, corrective actions and changes to manufacturing documents.
- Data for stability testing for several batches.
- Trend analyses including those for quality related complaints.

REVALIDATION

Re-validation is usually performed to the confirmation of initial validation for a periodic review. Revalidation is needed to ensure that changes in the process and / or in the process environment, whether intentional or unintentional, do not adversely affect process characteristics and product quality.

Revalidation may be divided into two broad categories:

➤ Revalidation after any change having a bearing on product quality.

➤ Periodic revalidation carried out at scheduled intervals.

REVALIDATION AFTER CHANGES

Revalidation must be performed on introduction of any changes affecting a manufacturing and / or standard procedure having a bearing on the established product performance characteristics. Such changes may include those in starting material, packaging material, manufacturing processes, equipment, in-process controls, manufacturing areas, or support systems (water, steam, etc.).

Every such change requested should be reviewed by a qualified validation group, which will decide whether it is significant enough to justify revalidation and if so, it extent.

Revalidation after changes may be based on the performance of the same tests and activities as those used during the original validation, including tests on sub processes and on the equipment concerned. Some typical changes which require revalidation include the following :-

➤ Changes in the starting materials(s). Changes in the physical properties, such as density, viscosity, particle size distribution, and crystal type and modification, of the active ingredients or excipients may affect the mechanical properties of the material; as a consequence, they may adversely affect the process or the product.

➢ Changes in the packaging material, e.g. replacing plastics by glass, may require changes in the packaging procedure and therefore affect product stability.

➢ Changes in the process, e.g. changes in mixing time, drying temperature and cooling regime, may affect subsequent process steps and product quality.

➢ Changes in equipment, including measuring instruments, may affect both the process and the product; repair and maintenance work, such as the replacement of major equipment components, may affect the process.

➢ Changes in the production area and support system, e.g. the rearrangement of manufacturing areas and / or support systems, may result in changes in the process. The repair and maintenance of support systems, e.g. the rearrangement of manufacturing areas and / or support systems, may result in changes in the process. The repair and maintenance of support systems, such as ventilation, may change the environmental conditions and, as a consequence, revalidation / requalification may be necessary, mainly in the manufacture of sterile products.

➢ Unexpected changes and deviations may be observed during self inspection or audit, or during the continuous trend analysis of process data.

PERIODIC REVALIDATION

It is well known that process changes may occur gradually even if experienced operators work correctly according to established methods. Similarly, equipment wear may also cause gradual changes. Consequently, revalidation at scheduled times is advisable even if no changes have been deliberately made.

The decision to introduce periodic revalidation should be based essentially on a review of historical data, i.e. data generated during in-process and finished product testing after the latest validation, aimed at verifying that the process is under control. During the data collected should be evaluated.

In some processes, such as sterilization, additional process testing is required to complement the historical data. The degree of testing required will be apparent from the original validation. Additionally, the following points should be checked at the time of a scheduled revalidation:

➤ Have any changes in master formula and methods, batch size, etc. occurred? If so, has their impact on the product been assessed?

➤ Have calibrations been made in accordance with the established programmed and time schedule?

➤ Has preventive maintenance been performed in accordance with the programme and time schedule?

➤ Have the standard operating procedures (SOPs) been properly updated?

➤ Have the SOPs been implemented?

➤ Have the cleaning and hygiene programmes been carried out?

➤ Have any changes been made in the analytical control methods?

8.9 ANALYTICAL METHOD VALIDATION

Validation of an analytical procedure is the process by which it is established, by laboratory studies, that the performance characteristics of the procedure meet the requirements for its intended use. All analytical methods that are intended to be used for analyzing any clinical samples will need to be validated. Validation of analytical methods is an essential but time - consuming activity for most analytical development laboratories. It is therefore important to understand the requirements of method validation in more detail and the options that are available to allow for optimal utilization of analytical resources in a development laboratory.

8.10 TYPES OF ANALYTICAL PROCEDURES TO BE VALIDATED

The validation of analytical procedures is directed to the four most common types of analytical procedures:

- Identification tests.
- Quantitative tests for impurities' content.
- Limit tests for the control of impurities.
- Quantitative tests of the active moiety in samples of drug substance or drug product or other selected component(s) in the drug product.

8.11 ICH/USP VALIDATION REQUIREMENTS & PARAMETERS

USP	ICH
Specificity	Specificity
Linearity and Range	Linearity
Accuracy	Range
Precision	Accuracy
Limit of Detection	PrecisionRepeatabilityIntermediate PrecisionReproducibility
Limit of Quantitation	Limit of Detection
Ruggedness	Limit of Quantitation
Robustness	

1.Accuracy: The International Convention on Harmonization (ICH) defines the accuracy of annalytical procedure as the closeness of agreement between the values that are accepted either as conventional true values or an accepted reference value and the value found.

For drug substance, accuracy may be defi ned by the application of the analytical procedure to an analyte of known purity (e.g., a reference standard).

For the drug product, accuracy will be determined by application of the analytical procedure to synthetic mixtures of the drug product components to which known amounts of analyte have been added within the range of the procedure.

Accuracy is usually reported as percent recovery by the assay (using the proposed analytical procedure) of known added amount of analyte in the sample or as the difference between the mean and the accepted true value together with the confidence intervals. The range for the accuracy limit should be within the linear range. Typical accuracy of the recovery of the drug substance is expected to be about 99 – 101%. Typical accuracy of the recovery of the drug product is expected to be about 98 – 102%. Values of accuracy of recovery data beyond this range need to be investigated as appropriate.

Precision

The precision of an analytical procedure expresses the closeness of agreement (degree of scatter) between a series of measurements obtained from multiple samples of the same homogeneous sample under prescribed conditions. Precision is usually investigated at three levels: repeatability, intermediate precision, and reproducibility.

Repeatability

Repeatability is a measure of the precision under the same operating conditions over a short interval of time, that is, under normal operating conditions of the analytical method with the same equipment. It is sometimes referred to as intra - assay precision.

The ICH recommends that repeatability be assessed using a minimum of nine determinations covering the specified range for the procedure (e.g., three concentrations/three replicates as in the accuracy experiment) or using a minimum of six determinations at 100% of the test concentration. Reporting of the standard deviation, relative standard deviation (coefficient of variation), and confidence interval is required.

Intermediate Precision: Intermediate precision is defined as the variation within the same laboratory. The extent to which intermediate precision needs to be established depends on the circumstances under which the procedure is intended to be used. Typical parameters that are investigated include day - to - day variation, analyst variation, and equipment variation. Depending on the extent of the study, the use of experimental design is encouraged. Experimental design will minimize the number of experiments that need to be performed.

Reproducibility: Reproducibility measures the precision between laboratories. This parameter is considered in the standardization of an analytical procedure To validate this characteristic, similar studies need to be performed at different laboratories using the same homogeneous sample lot and the same experimental design. In the case of method transfer between two laboratories, different approaches may be taken to achieve the successful transfer of the procedure.

Specificity

The ICH defines specificity as the ability to assess unequivocally an analyte in the presence of components that may be expected to be present. The specificity for an assay and impurity tests should be approached from two angles:

1. When impurities are available: The specificity of an assay method is determined by comparing test results from an analysis of sample containing the impurities, degradation products, or placebo ingredients with those obtained from an analysis of samples without the impurities, degradation products, or placebo ingredients.

2. If impurities are not available: Specificity may be demonstrated by comparing the test results of samples containing impurities or degradation products to a second well   characterized procedure or other validated analytical procedure (orthogonal method). This should include samples stored under relevant stress conditions (light, heat, humidity, acid/base hydrolysis and oxidation).

Detection Limit

The detection limit (DL) is a characteristic for the limit test only. It is the lowest amount of analyte in a sample that can be detected but not necessarily quantitated under the stated experimental conditions. The detection is usually expressed as the concentration of the analyte in the sample, for example, percentage, parts per million (ppm), or parts per billion (ppb).

There are several approaches to establish the detection limit. Visual evaluation may be used for non instrumental (e.g., solution color) and instrumental methods. In this case, the detection limit is determined by the analysis of a series of samples with known concentrations and establishing the minimum level at which the analyte can be reliably detected. For instrumental procedures that exhibit background noise, it is common to

compare measured signals from samples with known low concentrations of analyte with those of the blank samples. The minimum concentration at which the analyte can reliably be detected is established using an acceptable signal - to - noise ratio of 2 : 1 or 3 : 1. Presentation of relevant chromatograms is sufficient for justification of the detection limit.

Another approach estimates the detection limit from the standard deviation of the response

and the slope of the calibration curve. The standard deviation can be determined either from the standard deviation of multiple blank samples or from the standard deviation of the y intercepts of the regression lines done in the range of the detection limit.

$$DL = 3.3 \, \sigma/S$$

where σ is the standard deviation of the response and S is the slope of the calibration curve.

Quantitation Limit

The Quantitation Limit (QL) is a characteristic of quantitative assays for low levels of compounds in sample matrices, such as impurities in bulk drug substances and degradation products in finished pharmaceuticals. Quantitation Limit is defined as the concentration of related substance in the sample that will give a signal - to - noise ratio of 10 : 1. The quantitation limit of a method is affected by both the detector sensitivity and the accuracy of sample preparation at the low concentration of the impurities.

ICH recommends three approaches to the estimation of quantitation limit. The first approach is to evaluate it by visual evaluation and may be used for non instrumental methods and instrumental methods. Quantitation Limit is determined by the analysis of samples with known concentrations of analyte and by establishing the minimum level at which the analyte can be quantitated with acceptable accuracy and precision.

The second approach determines the signal - to - noise ratio by comparing measured signals from samples with known low concentrations of anlayte with those of blank samples. Quantitation Limit is the minimum concentration at which the analyte can be reliably quantifi ed at the signal - to - noise ratio of 10 : 1.The third approach estimates quantitation limit by the equation QL =10 σ/S . The value of σ may be estimated by (1) calculating the standard deviation of the responses obtained from the measurement of the analytical background response of an appropriate number of blank samples or (2) calculating the residual standard deviation of the regression line from the calibration curve using samples containing the analyte in the range of the quantitation limit .

Linearity

Linearity is defined as ability of the method to obtain test results which are directly proportional to the concentration of analyte in the sample within a given range. There are two general approaches for determining the linearity of the method. The first approach is to weigh different amounts of standard directly to prepare linearity solutions at different concentrations. Another approach is to prepare a stock solution of high concentration. Linearity is then demonstrated directly by dilution of the standard stock solution. Linearity is best evaluated by visual inspection of a plot of the signals as a function of analyte concentration. Subsequently, the variable data are generally used to calculate a regression line by the least - squares method. At least five concentration levels should be used. Under normal circumstances, linearity is acceptable with a coefficient of determination (r^2) of $\geq$ 0.997.

Range

The range of an analytical procedure is the interval between the upper and lower concentration of analyte in the sample for which it has been demonstrated that the analytical procedure has a suitable level of precision, accuracy, and linearity. The range is normally expressed in the same units as test results (e.g., percent, parts per million) obtained by the analytical procedure. For the assay of drug substance or finished drug product, it is normally recommended to have a range of 80 – 120% of the nominal concentration. For content uniformity, a normal range would cover 70 – 130% of the nominal concentration, unless a wider and more appropriate range (e.g., metered - dose inhalers) is justified. For dissolution testing, a normal range is ± 20% over the specified range. If the acceptance criterion for a controlled - release product covers a region from 20% after 1 h, and up to 90% after 24 h, the validated range would be 0 – 110% of the label claim. In this case, the lowest appropriate quantifiable concentration of analyte will be used as the lowest limit as 0% is not appropriate.

Robustness

Robustness of an analytical procedure is a measure of the analytical method to remain unaffected by small but deliberate variations in method parameters and provides an indication of its reliability during normal usage. The evaluation of robustness is normally considered during the development phase and depends on the type of procedure under study. It should show the reliability of an analysis with respect to deliberate variations in method parameters.

If measurements are susceptible to variations in analytical conditions, the analytical conditions should be suitably controlled or a precautionary statement should be included in the procedure. One consequence of the evaluation of robustness should be that a series of system suitability parameters (e.g., resolution test) is established to ensure that the validity of the analytical procedure is maintained whenever used.

Examples of typical variations are: stability of analytical solutions, extraction time.

In the case of liquid chromatography, examples of typical variations are influence of variations of pH in a mobile phase, influence of variations in mobile phase composition, Different columns (different lots and/or suppliers), temperature, flow rate.

Ruggedness

Ruggedness is the of reproducibility of the test results obtained for identical samples under normal (but variable) test conditions.

8.12 PROCESS OF ANALYTICAL METHOD VALIDATION

The typical process that is followed in an analytical method validation is chronologically listed below:

1. Planning and deciding on the method validation experiments

2. Writing and approval of method validation protocol

3. Execution of the method validation protocol

4. Analysis of the method validation data

5. Reporting the analytical method validation

6. Finalizing the analytical method procedure

The validation protocol should be numbered, signed and dated, and should contain as a minimum the following information

- Objectives, scope of coverage of the validation study.

- Validation team membership, their qualifications and responsibilities.

- Type of validation: prospective, concurrent, retrospective, re-validation.

- Number and selection of batches to be on the validation study.

- A list of all equipment to be used; their normal and worst case operating parameters.

- Outcome of IQ, OQ for critical equipment.

- Requirements for calibration of all measuring devices.

- Critical process parameters and their respective tolerances.

- Description of the processing steps: copy of the master documents for the product.

- Sampling points, stages of sampling, methods of sampling, sampling plans.

- Statistical tools to be used in the analysis of data.

- Training requirements for the processing operators.

- Validated test methods to be used in in-process testing and for the finished product.

- Specifications for raw and packaging materials and test methods.

- Forms and charts to be used for documenting results.

- Format for presentation of results, documenting conclusions and for approval of study results.

8.13 DOCUMENTATION

It is essential that the validation program is documented and that the documentation is properly maintained. Approval and release of the process for use in routine manufacturing should be based upon a review of all the validation documentation, including data from the equipment qualification, process performance qualification, and product/package testing to ensure compatibility with the process. For routine production, it is important to adequately record process details (e.g., time, temperature, equipment used) and to record any changes which have occurred. A maintenance log can be useful in performing failure investigations concerning a specific manufacturing lot. Validation data (along with specific test data) may also determine expected variance in product or equipment characteristics.

8.14 CLEANING VALIDATION

Introduction

Cleaning validation is a documented process that proves the effectiveness and consistency in cleaning a pharmaceutical production equipment. Validations of equipment cleaning procedures are mainly used in pharmaceutical industries to prevent cross contamination and adulteration of drug products. The prime purpose of validating a cleaning process is to ensure compliance with federal and other standard regulations. The most important benefit of conducting such a validation work is the identification and correction of potential problems previously unsuspected, which could compromise the safety, efficacy or quality of subsequent batches of drug product produced within the equipment. Pharmaceutical products and active pharmaceutical ingredients (APIs) can be contaminated by other pharmaceutical products or APIs, by cleaning agents, by micro-organisms or by other material (e.g., air-borne particles, dust, lubricants, raw materials, intermediates, auxiliaries). In many cases, the same equipment may be used for processing different products. To avoid contamination of the following pharmaceutical product, adequate cleaning procedures are essential. Cleaning procedures must strictly follow carefully established and validated methods of execution. This applies equally to the manufacture of pharmaceutical products and active pharmaceutical ingredients (APIs). In any case, manufacturing processes have to be designed and carried out in a way that contamination is reduced to an acceptable level. Cleaning Validation is documented evidence that an approved cleaning procedure will provide equipment which is suitable for processing of pharmaceutical products or active pharmaceutical ingredients (APIs).

Objective

The objectives of equipment cleaning and cleaning validation in an Active Pharmaceutical Ingredient (API) area are same as those in pharmaceutical production area. In both these areas efforts are necessary to prevent contamination of a future batch with the previous batch material.

The cleaning of 'difficult to reach' surface is one of the most important consideration in equipment cleaning validation. Equipment cleaning validation in an API facility is extremely important as cross contamination in one of the pharmaceutical dosage forms, will multiply the problem. Therefore, it is important to do a step-by-step evaluation of API process to determine the most practical and efficient way to monitor the effectiveness of the cleaning process. It is necessary to validate cleaning procedures for the following reasons.

1. It is a prime customer requirement since it ensures the purity and safety of the product.

2. It is a regulatory requirement in Active Pharmaceutical Ingredient product manufacture.

3. It also assures the quality of the process through an internal control and compliance.

8.15 TYPES OF CONTAMINATIONS

1. Cross contamination with active ingredients

Contamination of one batch of product with significant levels of residual active ingredients from a previous batch cannot be tolerated. In addition to the obvious problems posed by subjecting consumers or patients to unintended contaminants, potential clinically significant synergistic interactions between pharmacologically active chemicals are a real concern.

2. Contamination with unintended materials or compounds

While inert ingredients used in drug products are generally recognized as safe or have been shown to be safe for human consumption, the routine use, maintenance and cleaning of equipments provide the potential contamination with such items as equipment parts, lubricants, chemical cleaning agents and pieces of cleaning tools such as brushes and rags.

3. Microbiological contamination

Maintenance, cleaning and storage conditions may provide adventitious microorganisms with the opportunity to proliferate within the processing equipment.

8.16 GENERAL ASPECTS OF CLEANING VALIDATION

Personnel

Operators who perform cleaning routinely should be trained in the application of validated cleaning procedures. Training records should be available for all training carried out. It is difficult to validate a manual, i.e. an inherently variable/cleaning procedure. Therefore, operators carrying out manual cleaning procedures should be supervised at regular intervals.

Equipment

The design of the equipment should be carefully examined. Critical areas (those hardest to clean) should be identified, particularly in large systems that employ semi-automatic or fully automatic clean-in-place (CIP) systems. Dedicated equipment should be used for products which are difficult to remove (e.g., tarry or gummy residues in the bulk manufacturing), for equipment which is difficult to clean (e.g., bags for fluid bed dryers), or for products with a high safety risk (e.g., biologicals or products of high potency which may be difficult to detect below an acceptable limit).

Microbiological Aspects

The existence of conditions favourable to reproduction of micro organisms (e.g., moisture, temperature, crevices and rough surfaces) and the time of storage should be considered. The aim should be to prevent excessive microbial contamination. The period and when appropriate, conditions of storage of equipment before cleaning and the time between cleaning and equipment reuse, should form part of the validation of cleaning procedures. This is to provide confidence that routine cleaning and storage of equipment does not allow microbial proliferation.

8.17 CLEANING VALIDATION TECHNIQUES FOR MICROORGANISMS

1. Swab Method

2. Surface Rinse Method

3. RODAC Plate Method

4. Limulus Amoebocyte Lysate Method

5. ATP Bioluminescence Method

1. Swab Method

After cleaning the equipment, product contact surfaces could be swabbed to evaluate surface cleanliness. Swabs used should be compatible with the active ingredients and should not interfere with the assay. They should not cause any degradation of the compound. The solvent used for swabbing should provide good solubility for the compound and should not encourage degradation.

Advantages: Most common method used with selective media to isolate directly different microbial populations.

Disadvantages: Recovery may not be reproducible & quantitative.

2.Surface Rinse Method

Sampling and testing of rinse samples for residual active ingredient is a commonly adopted method to evaluate cleanliness. This is a fairly convenient method in many cases and requires control over the solvent used for rinsing, the contact time and the mixing involved. The solvent used should be selected based on the solubility of the active ingredient and should either simulate a subsequent batch of product or at least provide adequate solubility.

Advantages: Higher counts obtained than swab method and better overall assessment possible.

Disadvantages: Entire surface evaluated, microbial population must be detached and membrane filtration necessary to obtain countable numbers.

3. Replicate Organism Direct Agar Contact Plate Method:

All samples will be collected on RODAC Plates. Surfaces, such as walls, floors, and ceilings should be dry and have been sanitized within twelve hours of being sampled. Items such as cages and sipper tubes should be sampled close to five minutes after being disinfected. Two different techniques will be used for obtaining samples, depending on the sample site. These techniques include:

• **Flat Surfaces:** Gently press the rounded agar surface of the plate to the sample surface. Use a rolling motion, with a light uniform pressure, to ensure that the entire surface of the agar will contact the sample surface. Avoid pulling or sweeping the agar surface over the sample area, as this will destroy the agar surface, thereby rendering plate unusable.

• **Irregular Surfaces:** A sterile, cotton-tipped swab is moistened with sterile water and swabbed over such surfaces and into the corners of equipment. In the case of sipper tubes, the swab should be passed into and out of the tube three times. For other irregular surfaces, the swab should be rubbed over a surface area roughly the same size as the base of the RODAC Plate three times in an opposite direction between each successive stroke. Following sampling, the swab head should be gently rotated over the surface of the agar three times, again rolling in opposite direction between each successive stroke.

The RODAC Plates are placed upside down in the incubator located in the lab. The incubator should always be set on 36.7°C. After a 24 hour period, the plates are observed for growth. After 48 hours, the plates are removed from the incubator and the colonies counted using the electronic colony counter pen. After results are recorded, the plates are placed in a Bio-Hazard bag and disposed.

Results – The following system will be used to rate the results:

• 0-5 colonies: None or Very slight colonies (considered excellent)

• 6-15 colonies: Slight (considered good)

• 16-30 colonies: Moderate (borderline acceptable)

• 31-50 colonies: Significant (poor)

• >50 colonies: Heavy (unacceptable)

Advantages: Direct growth on media in contact plate is convenient, neutralizers may be included in media & different media may be used.

Disadvantages: Only applicable to surfaces that are smooth & have low counts.

4.Limulus Amoebocyte Lysate Method

This technique was widely used in the biopharmaceutical industry. The LAL test is performed by adding aliquots of sample or test materials to small quantities of a lysate preparation, followed by incubation at 37°C for 1 hour. The presence of endotoxins causes gel formation of the lysate material.

Advantages: Rapid, sensitive, quantitative measure of bacterial endotoxin levels.

Disadvantages: Indirect measurement of high numbers of gram-negative bacteria only.

5.ATP Bioluminescence Method

This type of analysis usually uses ATP-bioluminescence. The bioluminescence technique is an increasingly important alternative to classical microbiological methods. A defined surface area is wiped with a special swab and in the presence of magnesium ions, The extracted ATP is converted into light by means of a luciferin-luciferase enzymatic system. The result is available within a few minutes.

Advantages: Rapid, highly accurate & reliable method.

Disadvantages: Suitable for microbial counts in the range of 10^4 to 10^8 organisms as insufficiently sensitive for low microbial counts.

8.18 CLEANING VALIDATION TECHNIQUES FOR CONTAMINANTS OR PREVIOUS PRODUCT RESIDUES

1. Swab method
2. Rinse solvent method
3. Conductivity testing
4. Placebo method

1.Swab method

Swabbing is commonly used to sample the surface of cleaned materials. The swab is then placed in a sample vial and sent to the Quality Control lab for analysis. Proper analytical technique is essential in order to evaluate the effectiveness of cleaning techniques.

2. Rinse method:

Analysis of rinse water for residual cleaning agents or process materials is an essential component of cleaning validation. Insuring that the sample is not contaminated requires vigilance and properly following the relevant SOP's.

3. Conductivity method

The variation in conductivity of rinsed solvent indicates the cleaning efficiency. This method commonly employed for reactors, centrifuges and piping between large equipments.

4. Placebo method

Placebo is an inert material in which contaminants are dissolved or dispersed. Placebo method should be used in conjugation with Rinse or Swab method. Assurance found to be less when compared to other methods. It is not suitable for contaminants having higher particle size.

8.19 DETERGENTS

The efficiency of cleaning procedures for the removal of detergent residues should be evaluated. Acceptable limits should be defined for levels of detergent after cleaning. Ideally, there should be no residues detected. The possibility of detergent breakdown should be considered when validating cleaning procedures.

Detergents selection

Detergent should be easily removable.

The composition of the detergent should be known.

The possibility of detergent breakdown and detergent removal should be demonstrated.

Acceptable limits should be defined for detergent residues after cleaning.

8.20 ANALYTICAL METHODS

The analytical methods should be validated before the Cleaning Validation Study is carried out.

The analytical methods used to detect residuals or contaminants should be specific for the substance to be assayed and provide a sensitivity that reflects the level of cleanliness determined to be acceptable by the company.

The analytical methods should be challenged in combination with the sampling methods used, to show that the contaminants can be recovered from the equipment surface and to show the level of recovery as well as the consistency of recovery.

8.21 ANALYSIS OF CLEANING VALIDATION SAMPLES

There are many analytical techniques available that can be used in cleaning validation. But choosing the appropriate analytical tool depends on a variety of factors. The most important factor is to determine the specifications or parameters to be measured. The limit should always be established prior to the selection of the analytical tool.

1. Analysis of anionic and cationic surfactants is done by HPLC and Capillary electrophoresis (CE),where as amphoteric surfactants are analysed by HPLC and Evaporate light scattering detector.

2. Capillary electrophoresis can be used for many different types of analysis, viz; separation, detection and determination of sodium lauryl sulphate in cationic, anionic and non-ionic surfactant.

3. Micellar electro kinetic capillary chromatography is used for the separation of non-ionic alkyl phenol polyoxyethylene type surfactants.

4. Total organic carbon is used for the analysis of detergents, endotoxins, biological media and poly ethylene glycol.

5. Ion chromatography can be used for the analysis of inorganic, organic and surfactants present in the cleaners.

6. Thin layer chromatography is widely used for the qualitative determination of surfactants.

7. Atomic absorption spectroscopy is used for the determination of inorganic contaminants.

8. Portable mass spectrometer can be used to detect ultra sensitive measurements and identification of the residue.

8.22 ACCEPTANCE CRITERIA

Carry-over of product residues should meet defined criteria, for example the most stringent of the following three criteria:

Chemical

(a) No more than 0.1% of the normal therapeutic dose of any product will appear in the maximum daily dose of the following product.

(b) No more than 10 ppm of any product will appear in another product.

Visual

No quantity of residue should be visible on the equipment after cleaning procedures are performed.

(a) No quantity of residue should be visible on the equipment after cleaning procedures are performed. Spiking studies should determine the concentration at which most active ingredients are visible.

(b) For certain allergenic ingredients, penicillins, cephalosporins or potent steroids and cytotoxics, the limit should be below the limit of detection by best available analytical methods.

Microbiological limit

Total aerobic microbial count	- NMT 1000 cfu/g
Total combined Yeast and mold count	- NMT 100 cfu/g
Absence of USP indicator organisms i.e.	- E.coli
	- S. aureus
	- Salmonella species

8.23 CURRENT APPROACHES IN DETERMINING THE ACCEPTANCE LIMITS FOR CLEANING VALIDATION

Acceptance limits for pharmaceutical manufacturing operation.

1. Approach 1 (Dose criterion)

Not more than 0.001 of minimum daily dose of any product will appear in the maximum daily dose of another product.

Milligrams of active ingredient = I x K x M in product A permitted per J x L 4 inch^2 swab area

I = 0.001 of the smallest strength of product A manufactured per day expressed as mg/day and based on the number of milligrams of active ingredient.

J = Maximum number of dosage units of product B per day

K = Number of dosage units per batch of final mixture of product B

L = Equipment surface in common between product A & B expressed as square inches.

M= 4 $inch^2$/swab.

2. Approach 2 (10 ppm criterion)

Any active ingredient can be present in a subsequently manufactured product at a maximum level of 10 ppm.

Milligrams of active ingredient = R x S x U in product A permitted per T 4 $inch^2$ swab area

R = 10mg active ingredient of product A in one kg of product B

S = Number of kilograms per batch of final mixture of product B

T = Equipment surface in common between product A & B expressed as square inches.

U = 4 $inch^2$/swab.

3. Approach 3 (Visually clean criterion)

No quantity of residue should be visible on the equipment after cleaning procedures are performed.

8.24 DOCUMENTATION

Cleaning Validation Protocol is required laying down the procedure on how the cleaning process will be validated. It should include the following:

The objective of the validation process

Responsibilities for performing and approving the validation study,

Description of the equipment to be used,

The interval between the end of production and the beginning of the cleaning procedures,

Cleaning procedures to be used for each product and each manufacturing system

The number of cleaning cycles to be performed consecutively,

Any routine monitoring requirement,

Sampling procedures, including the rationale for why a certain sampling method is used,

Clearly defined sampling locations,

Data on recovery studies where appropriate,

Analytical methods:

The acceptance criteria, including the rationale for setting the specific limits,

The Cleaning Validation Protocol should be formally approved by the plant management, to ensure that aspects relating to the work defined in the protocol, for example personnel resources, are known and accepted by the management. Quality Assurance should be involved in the approval of protocols and reports. The cleaning process should be documented in an SOP.

8.25 STANDARD CLEANING PROCEDURES

Standard cleaning procedures for each piece of equipment and process should be prepared. It is vital that the equipment design is evaluated in detail in conjunction with the product residues which are to be removed, the available cleaning agents and cleaning techniques, when determining the optimum cleaning procedure for the equipment.

Cleaning procedures should be sufficiently detailed to remove the possibility of any inconsistencies during the cleaning process. Following parameters are to be considered during cleaning procedures.

A. Equipment Parameters to be evaluated

1. Identification of the equipment to be cleaned

2. 'Difficult to clean' areas

3. Property of materials

4. Ease of disassembly

5. Mobility

B. Residues to be cleaned

1. Cleaning limits

2. Solubility of the residues

3. Length of campaigns

C. Cleaning agent parameters to be evaluated

1. Preferable materials that are normally used in the process

2. Detergents available (as a general guide, minimal use of detergents recommended unless absolutely required)

3. Solubility properties

4. Environmental considerations

5. Health and safety considerations

D. Cleaning techniques to be evaluated

1. Manual cleaning

2. CIP (Clean-in-place)

3. COP (Clean-out-of-place)

4. Semi automatic procedures

5. Automatic procedures

6. Time considerations

7. Number of cleaning cycles

8.26 VALIDATION REPORT

A validation report is necessary to present the results and conclusions and secure approval of the study. The report should include the following information:

1. References to all the procedures followed to clean the samples and tests.

2. Physical and analytical test results or references for the same, as well as any pertinent observations.

3. Conclusions regarding the acceptability of the results, and the status of the procedures being validated.

4. Any recommendations based on the results or relevant information obtained during the study including revalidation practices if applicable.

5. Review of any deviations from the protocol.

6. When it is unlikely that further batches of the product will be manufactured for a period of time, it is advisable to generate reports on a batch by batch basis until such time.

7. The report should conclude an appropriate level of verification subsequent to validation.

ESSAY QUESTIONS

1. Write the various types of process validation?

2. a. Write a notes on the concept and importance of Validation?

   b. Write a note on cleaning validation?

3. Write the requirements & parameters for analytical method validation?

4. Write the sampling procedure and acceptance criteria for cleaning validation?

5. Write the Phases of Process Validation ?

6. Write about Process Validation protocol and Process Validation Report?

7. Write about analytical method Validation protocol?

SHORT ANSWER QUESTIONS

1. Write the Process of analytical method validation?

2. Write the sampling procedure for cleaning validation?

3. Write the acceptance criteria for cleaning validation?

4. Write the Objective and general aspects of cleaning validation?

5. Write the sampling techniques for microorganisms in Cleaning validation?

6. Write the sampling techniques for contaminants or previous product residues in Cleaning validation?

7. Write about various analytical techniques for analysis of cleaning validation samples?

8. Write about Prospective Validation?

9. Which circumstances favours the concurrent validation?

10. Write the essential elements for Retrospective Validation

11. Which aspects should be considered at the time of a scheduled revalidation?

12. Write about Detection Limit and Quantitation Limit?

REFERENCES / BIBLIOGRAPHY

1. Yie Chien, Novel drug delivery systems, Informa Healthcare

2. Prescott,Novel Drug Delivery and Its Therapeutic Application, Johns Hopkins press.

3. L. Lachman, H.A, Lieberman and J.L. Kanig, Theory & Practice of industrial pharmacy by, Lea & Febieger, Philadelphia Latest Edn.

4: Novel Drug Delivery Systems For Gene-Targeted RNA Interference: Application of RNAi for Cancer Gene Therapy by Randy Adachi

5. Leon Shargel Isadore Kanfer, Generic Drug Product Development, Solid Oral Dosage Forms, Marcel Dekker.

6. Novel Drug Delivery Systems For Gene-Targeted RNA Interference: Application of RNAi for Cancer Gene Therapy by Randy Adachi

7. Lippincott Williams and Wilkins, Remington Pharmaceutical Sciences

8. E.A Rawlkins, Bentley's Text Book of Pharmaceutics, Elbs publ

9. HC Ansel, Introduction to Pharmaceutical Dosage forms

10. S.H. Willing, M.M Tucherman and W.S. Hitchings IV, Good Manufacturing Practices for Pharmaceuticals: A Plan for Total Quality Control, Marcel Dekker, Inc., New York

11. Gilbert S. Banker and Christopher T Rhodes, Modern Pharmaceutics, IVth ed, marcel dekker, usa, 2005.

12. Good Design Practices for GMP Pharmaceutical Facilities (Drugs and the Pharmaceutical Sciences) by Andrew Signore and Terry Jacobs, Marcel Dekker

13. Robert. A. Nash, Pharmaceutical Process Validation, 3rd Ed Marcel Dekker, 2003.

14. Good Manufacturing Practices – Schedule M Read with The Drugs And Cosmetic Rules 1945.

15. M.E. Aulton, Pharmaceuitcs- The science of Dosage form Design 2nd ed.

16. Analytical Chemistry in a GMP Environment: A Practical Guide - Hardcover (Apr. 17, 2000) by James M. Miller